YOGA FOR REGULAR GUYS

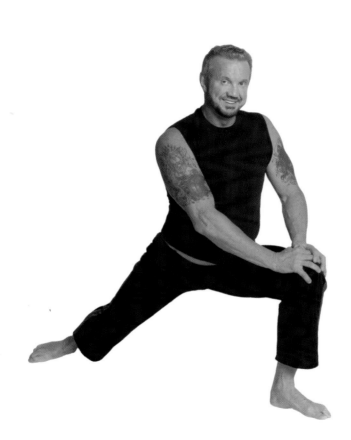

DEDICATION

I want to dedicate this book to a bro who I thought would never be caught dead doing yoga. His name is George Hyder. George was a wild man, the kind of man that guys wanted to be and women—well, they all loved George. He was an in-your-face boot-camp Marine sergeant personal trainer. You would never have guessed in a million years that George Hyder was also a yogi, but he was. I'll never forget the day he came up to me with that strong South Carolina accent and said: "DDP, I was watching earlier, and I've got to know—when did you start doing yoga?" I was amazed that he knew what I was doing. I actually thought someone had put him up to it as a rib, but then he started going into all these one-legged standing positions, and I was truly blown away. He went on about how good yoga was for core strength and how it could really keep me from getting injured in the ring. I immediately asked George about personally training me in yoga, and he helped me take my yoga to a whole new level. He showed me that if guys like us were doing it, then there was a whole world out there just waiting to get the word from a Regular Guy.

Thank you, George. You are always with me, bro, and I dedicate this book to you. May you rest in peace, my brother.

Copyright © 2005 by AuthorScape, Inc.
Text Copyright © 2005 by Dallas Page

All rights reserved. No part of this book may be reproduced in any form without written permission from the publisher.

Library of Congress Cataloging in Publication Number: 2005925096

ISBN: 1-59474-079-8

Printed in China

Typeset in Meta Normal and Conduit ITC

Photography by Maximo Morrone
Photo credits: p. 162, photo by Peter King; p. 172, photos by Ross Foreman; pp. 164, 175, photos by Hexphoto.com; p. 173, photo courtesy of Warner Brothers

Distributed in North America by Chronicle Books
85 Second Street
San Francisco, CA 94105

10 9 8 7 6 5 4 3 2 1

Yoga for Regular Guys is an AUTHORSCAPE BOOK PRODUCTION
Designed by Laurie Dolphin and Allison Meierding, Laurie Dolphin Design

Quirk Books
215 Church Street
Philadelphia, PA 19106
www.quirkbooks.com

YOGA FOR REGULAR GUYS

THE BEST DAMN WORKOUT ON THE PLANET!

By DIAMOND DALLAS PAGE

With Dr. Craig Aaron

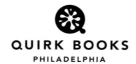

QUIRK BOOKS

PHILADELPHIA

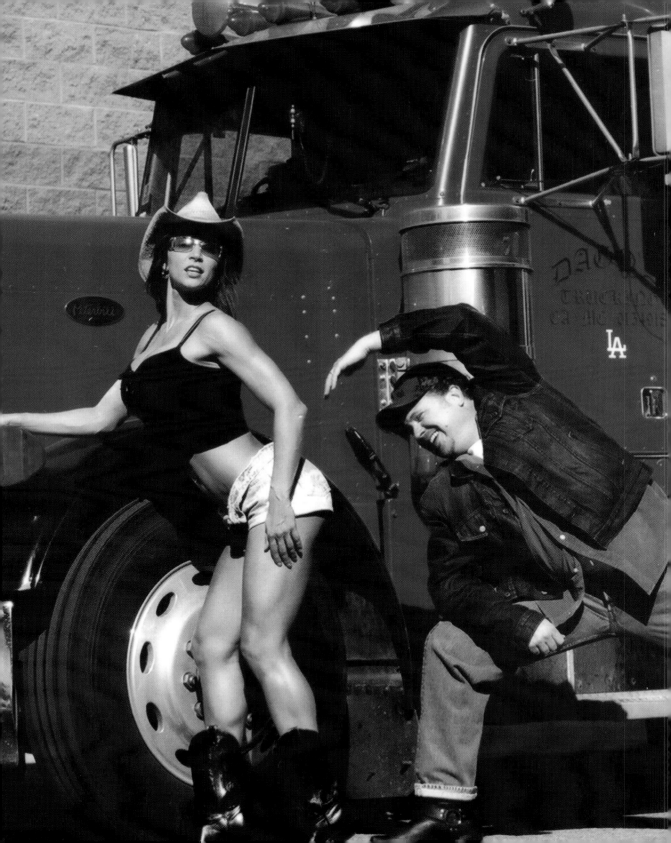

➤ CONTENTS

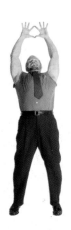

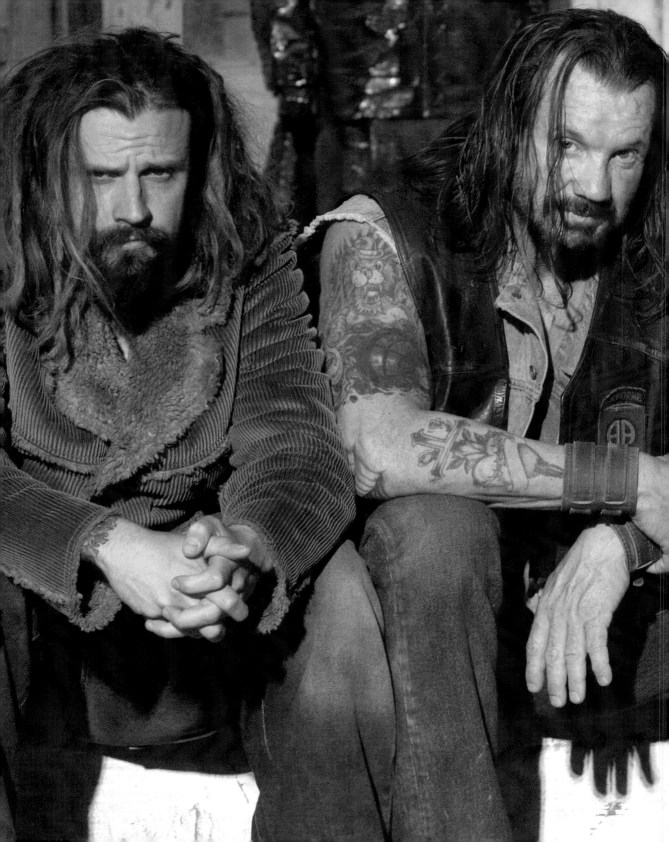

FOREWORD

Yoga?

Give me a f***ing break!

If you're anything like me, you know that even the sound of the word *yoga* will get you a sarcastic roll of the eyeballs and a loud Bronx cheer. I mean, come on—YOGA! Yeah, sure, let's all sit around cross-legged, chanting to our inner peace while sucking down on wheat germ smoothies and feeling at one with the f***ing universe. I mean, this is what yoga is all about, right? This is girlie-man hippie crap, right?

Well, that's the way I always saw it. That is, until Diamond Dallas Page explained *Yoga for Regular Guys* to me. Hey, I figured if *this* guy thought yoga was a badass workout, maybe— and I emphasize *maybe*—there might be something to this New Age voodoo.

Truthfully, if it weren't for the fact that this DDP guy is built like a block of granite and could most certainly crush my skull, I would have laughed my ass off at the thought of doing that Down Dog/Warrior One shit. I mean, really: Only spiritual head-cases need to twist like a pretzel for fun, right?

But one day I agreed to give it a shot. What did I have to lose?

On a hot summer afternoon I roll out my mat and get ready for action. The first thing DDP says is that he's going to teach me how to breathe. Listen, buddy, I think to myself, I might not know how to whoop ass in the squared circle, but I know how to f***ing *breathe*! But like I said, he's a big guy, so I decided to go along with this breathing deal. After about fifteen minutes of trying not to laugh, I realize this ain't exactly what I thought it was. This shit is *difficult* . . . seriously. Pretty soon, I wasn't laughing anymore. I was *feeling the burn*, as they say. I'm trying to activate muscles that have been in a coma for well . . . well, forever, really.

To make a long story short, Yoga for Regular Guys *works*, and trust me, it ain't what you think. It's a total body, kick-ass workout that whips you into shape. Think of it as yoga meets old school calisthenics by way of slow burn isometric movements. Translation: something fun to kick that flabby-ass body of yours into shape! Let's face it folks, DDP is the new Jack LaLanne for the hardcore, cynical, regular-guy "I'm-too-cool-for-that" generation. Here's my advice to you: Put down the doughnuts, pick up this book, and get with the YRG program . . . or else!

—ROB ZOMBIE
Los Angeles, California

◄ I knew I could never get RZ to have his picture taken doing YRG, so this is a picture of RZ and me on the set of *Devil's Rejects*. —DDP

INTRODUCTION

WHO IS THE REGULAR GUY?

If you picked this book up, you're most likely one of them. Or else you're close enough to one to know that the only yoga book you'll ever get him to read would be written by a pro wrestler. Regular Guys are everywhere: They're athletes, CEOs, cops, firemen, construction workers, bartenders, and lawyers; well, I may need to get back to you on lawyers, but I think you get the point.

YOGA FOR REGULAR GUYS . . . YOU'RE KIDDING, RIGHT?

Ask a Regular Guy if he does yoga, and he'll probably say, "I wouldn't be caught *dead* doing that crap—it's for girls."

I know, because that was my exact response when I was first introduced to yoga six years ago. If at any point in my life someone told me that I'd be writing a book about the benefits of yoga, I would have said, "I'm sorry. You must have me confused with another six-foot-four-inch, two-hundred-thirty-five-pound pro wrestler who beats people up with steel folding chairs." (Incidentally, in case you don't know me, I'm a professional wrestler, not a chaplain in a funeral home.)

So whatever made me, DDP, try yoga? Well, at the age of forty-two, the doctors said my professional wrestling career was over. I was on the top of the world at that time, in one main event after the other. But in 1998 I ruptured my L4/L5 disc so badly that I lost just about all flexibility in my lower back. I could barely bend over, never mind wrestle. You can say what you want about professional wrestling, but when it comes to getting bounced around in the ring, you can't *fake* gravity.

I remember that night like it was last night. I was battling the NWO (New World Order), and my opponent was Kevin Nash (6'10", 335 lbs.). The problem with facing the NWO was, you didn't just face one of them—you faced *all* of them. Near the end of the match, Scott Hall (6'6", 285 lbs.)

rolled into the ring and blasted me with the World Championship title belt. Then Kevin picked me up on his shoulders like I was a child and power-bombed me flat down on my back for the win—dirty cheatin' bastards.

When I hit the mat, my body jackknifed, and it felt like my spine had broken in half. Nash didn't mean to hurt me; it's not like we were playing checkers out there. He actually laid me out as flat as he ever had, but this time, it hurt like hell. It wasn't just that fall; it was an accumulation of all the falls I had taken in the ring over the years, like the one I just described, along with years of getting splattered by guitars, steel chairs, and garbage cans, that finally caught up with me.

You see, even though most athletes retire in their mid- to late thirties, I didn't get into the ring until I was thirty-five, and at forty-two, I was just hitting my stride. This Regular Guy was pretty bummed out.

But one day, while I was laid up in bed with my back injury, I noticed my wife, Kimberly, coming upstairs from one of her workouts. She was absolutely soaked in sweat. When she told me she was practicing yoga, I thought for sure she was pulling my leg. But she insisted that yoga sessions offered her a great physical workout, and also simply made her feel rejuvenated. She was absolutely certain that yoga could help me rehabilitate my back, and she asked me to start practicing with her.

Aside from the obvious worry of my buddies finding out I was off looking like Grasshopper in *Kung Fu,* I was concerned that yoga could worsen my condition. However, Kimberly convinced me that, because I was injured, I could work at my own pace. So my attorney sent over a confidentiality agreement, which Kimberly signed, and I decided to give it a shot.

WHAT IS YOGA?

Guys, I'm not bullshitting when I say that in my entire life I've never experienced a more profound and gratifying workout as those I've had in yoga.

The word *yoga* actually means "union," and the practice of yoga began about five thousand years ago. The old school yoga guys were called *yogis*—and I don't mean Yogi Bear. These yogis were looking for different ways to exercise, breathe, eat, sing, think, and meditate in order to live vibrant, healthy lives. They even talked about celibacy, but I'm not buyin' that part. (I'm sure there were some yoga-babes *somewhere*.) Their goal was to put together a lifestyle program that created a perfect balance of body, mind, and spirit. They devised an incredible exercise system called *Hatha yoga*, which produces flexibility, strength, balance, stamina, and mental focus.

To me, the word *yoga* means balance: having a good, healthy balance in your entire life. But also, on the physical level, I'm talking about the balance of strength and flexibility. Both are important. A lot of guys are strong, but they have little or no flexibility. Trust me when I tell you this is *not* a good thing. To me, flexibility means youth. The more flexible you are, the younger you feel, and the less chance you have for injury.

Over the years, many different styles of yoga were developed, but the three main systems are *Iyengar yoga*, which is very biomechanical and therapeutic in nature; *Ashtanga yoga*, which is athletic, acrobatic, and ridiculously challenging; and *Viniyoga*, which is a more moderate program that is based on the needs of each individual practitioner.

My favorite kind of yoga, besides Yoga for Regular Guys, is "power yoga," which is the Americanized version of the Ashtanga style. The term *power yoga* was originally coined by an incredible yoga-lady by the name of Beryl Bender Birch in the early 1980s. She called it *power yoga* in order to draw athletes into her Ashtanga Yoga classes. But a guy named Brian Kest really took power yoga and ran with it. He took the very challenging Ashtanga style and made it more accessible for those with a more Western body type. I originally learned yoga from Brian's videotapes. His system is really good, but the Regular Guy might have a tough time relating to the spiritual stuff—you know, meditating and finding your inner-self stuff.

I've had the pleasure of working out in Brian's classes—he's a very cool dude—on many occasions, and I really enjoy them (lots of yoga-babes), but I wanted to do something a little different. That's why I decided to do this book.

WHAT IS YOGA FOR REGULAR GUYS?

You see, most serious yogis are more about "namaste," a spiritual greeting that means "I honor the divine light within you." But Yoga for Regular Guys (YRG) is a little more "T & A" (which is the Regular Guy greeting to a hot yoga-babe that means "I honor the gorgeous round things that God, or possibly your plastic surgeon, has given you").

The yoga I'm talking about is not a religion. We won't be meditating or chanting "Om," and no one is going to be asked to put on a pair of footie pajamas. (That is, unless you're into that type of thing.) It's all about the *workout* and getting back to where you need to be with your health and fitness. YRG will challenge you, get you in great shape, and chill you out all at the same time. In fact, if I were allowed to do only one type of exercise for the rest of my life, I swear to God, I would choose yoga because of its broad range of benefits.

With this book, we've taken yoga to a whole new level. YRG is the perfect fusion of old-school calisthenics and core stability training, along with the hot new concept of slow-motion isometric strength training. We've taken a few time-tested calisthenics, like push-ups and squats, and we've turned up the heat by slowing them down into a slow-motion burn. This combination will add strength and endurance to anything you do. We will incorporate the isometric aspect into YRG by teaching you how to engage your muscles in every position for the entirety of the workout. You will be training your core from start to finish, and we've added some super core strength exercises if you're up for the challenge. Power yoga is our base, which is where this entire workout comes from. We've just modified it to make YRG more guy-friendly. This workout is the Bomb!

You see, yoga exercise works a lot like chiropractic and massage therapy. They all increase blood flow *and* nerve flow to every part of your body. So all of those locked-up and closed-off areas will be receiving more oxygen and healing life force than they probably had since you were a kid! And yoga releases enough tension in your body that it can make almost any therapeutic treatment, such as chiropractic care or massage, much more effective.

I still find myself amazed at what my body is capable of doing now after all I've put it through. For instance, you may not believe this, but I've written this entire introduction while standing on my head. Well, that may be stretching it, but believe me when I say that yoga not only allowed me to recover quickly, it has been proven helpful in preventing injuries as well.

MEET THE YOGA-DOC

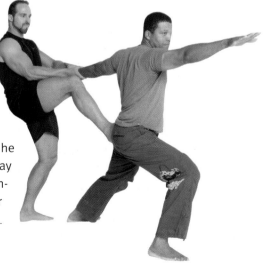

Shortly after being introduced to yoga through the Brian Kest videos, I met Dr. Craig Aaron, a sports chiropractor, trainer, and certified yoga instructor who has trained, among others, Georgia Tech's basketball and tennis teams, members of the Senior PGA tour, as well as many superstars of the NFL, MLB, and major college football teams. The "Yoga-Doc" (at left in this picture), as he is now known, not only taught me more about the day-to-day benefits of practicing yoga (after he signed that confidentiality agreement), but also became my tag-team partner in the writing and development of this entire YRG program. You'll see his pointers throughout the book.

THE BENEFITS OF YOGA; A.K.A. WHAT'S IN IT FOR ME?

Look, I know most Regular Guys are not professional wrestlers. Most Regular Guys don't get beaten up for a living. (That is, unless you're the sort of Regular Guy who thinks he's getting away with reading the introduction to this book and putting it back on the shelf.) But we all have things in common. As time passes, our bodies all become stiffer, regardless of our line of work. We lose flexibility and we lose strength. A lot of guys go to the gym to stay bulked up, but they do nothing about their flexibility. It's a rut that the Regular Guy doesn't have to be in. I am a walking, living example of someone who has beaten the hell out his body for years and still feels great after achieving flexibility through yoga. Flexibility, my friends, is youth.

Another benefit is time. I meet so many people who say, "I'm too busy to work out. I just don't have the time." My question to them is always, "Do you have twenty minutes?" Everyone can spare twenty minutes, and that's all you'll need to do the workouts in this book. There's a reason yoga has been around for five thousand years. It's the best use of your time, and it works. Most Regular Guys don't have time to lift weights three or four days a week, work on cardiovascular, and also manage to fit some flexibility/stretching into their routine. And for those guys who are asking themselves, "What about all that jumping up and down I do watching the football game?," get real. This isn't a "get rich quick scheme" or a guarantee that you'll go from looking like George of the Jungle to George Clooney, but the fact is, yoga is the most efficient five-thousand-year-old exercise system on the planet.

Many people do yoga just for its ability to reduce stress without beating the crap out of their knees and backs the way that hiking, jogging, or running does. But wait, there's more! Yoga does a lot more than just relax your mind for a little while. There has been an incredible amount of new research that points to yoga as a major player in normalizing blood pressure and improving sleep patterns, and it can also help people be less dependent on medication.

Today, I practice yoga because it's the best damn workout you can do for your body and your mind. It really helps you focus in every aspect of your life, and you can do it at your own pace. When I first started doing yoga, most of the guys in the locker room or in the gym wondered what the hell I was doing. As time went by, the same guys would watch my flexibility and strength increase, and one by one they would all start asking questions.

I told them the same thing I plan on teaching you in this book. In short, if you commit twenty minutes three or four days a week to your practice, you can receive the benefits of increased strength, flexibility, cardiovascular endurance, muscle tone, oxygen uptake, and improved confidence. YRG exercises also improve your posture, increase your energy levels, reduce stress, help you sleep better, and burn fat! That's right, you can lose weight, get into shape, and feel better by putting in three or four days a week! Now if the twenty-minute program really gets you charged and you want to move forward, this book will show you how to increase your workouts to thirty minutes and even forty-five minutes. We've also added five- and ten-minute routines just to get you energized in the middle of the day. You will notice that proper breathing while doing the YRG workout increases blood flow, which can give you instant energy.

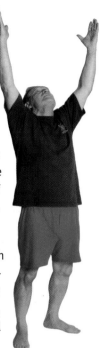

Yoga is definitely becoming mainstream in the United States, but it has yet to reach the Regular Guy. And that's not going to happen until the Regular Guy has someone teaching him whom he can relate to. I am that guy. I spent half of my life in nightclubs, drinking and throwing parties that would have made Caligula blush. Hell, I graduated from Regular Guy University, *summa cum laude*. I'm a professional wrestler! So you can trust me on this.

ALL RIGHT, I'M GAME: WHAT DO I HAVE TO DO?

You might be thinking, "How much equipment do I have to buy to do this yoga thing?" Once you know what you're doing, all you need is *you*. If you want to see your results right in front of you, I suggest you get a heart monitor to help you stay in your fat-burning zone, a yoga mat, some shorts, a T-shirt, and your bare feet. And, you can do yoga anywhere: at home, in a hotel room, anywhere—no gym membership required.

First, we'll teach you about breathing properly and how important it is for you to move and breathe in a specific way to get the most out of your YRG workouts.

Next, you'll learn your specific target heart rate and how to monitor your heart rate during these workouts so that you can maximize your cardiovascular and fat-burning benefits. Regular Guys like to see results right in front of their eyes. You guys will be blown away when you see just how high your heart rate will actually go while doing the simplest positions. It may all sound pretty complicated, but I promise that we will use the KISS method of teaching: "Keep It Stupidly Simple" and very easy to follow.

The twenty-minute program will get you moving and build your flexibility and endurance. I'm going to give you basic moves to get you started, and I won't have you twisted up like a pretzel. As you continue your workouts, you will notice that the tougher yoga positions will be the ones that give you the most benefit. However, even if you stick with the more basic program, you will keep getting stronger, more flexible, more centered, leaner, and healthier.

OH, AND ONE MORE BENEFIT I HAVEN'T MENTIONED YET . . .

Let's see: more relaxed, less fatigued, better range of motion, increased nerve flow and blood flow to all parts of the body. That sounds like a prescription for a better sex life to me! You gotta know, it's all about the flow. Guys, the couple that does yoga together has better sex—go figure. (For starters *she's* more flexible, if you get my drift.)

And if you're single . . . *fuhgeddaboudit*! I can't think of a better place to meet women who are in, or already on their way to being in, great shape with great, flexible bodies than in the yoga studio.

Come to think of it, I bet the reason all the Regular Guys who've been doing yoga for years have never smartened the rest of us up is because they want to keep all those hot yoga-babes for themselves.

So, bro, what are you waiting for? DDP is ready to take you back where you belong. It's all about feeling better today than you did yesterday, right? So let's do it! What the hell, give it a shot!

A WORD FROM THE WIFE

When I first tried to get Dallas to try yoga as a way to help his back pain, I was surprised by his reaction. He didn't even want to try it! Page is famously open-minded and receptive, but he turned me down FLAT! "That stuff's for chicks," he grumbled. But one day, his lower back was feeling particularly stiff. After some gentle cajoling, I got him to join me downstairs.

After twenty minutes, he was sweating, straining, and grunting through the poses like it was football practice. In extended side angle pose, I could see him glancing over at me, attempting to go as deeply into it as I was. "No, honey," I chuckled. "You're supposed to kinda just relax and breathe. You don't have to work so hard at it." But his competitive nature wouldn't have it. At the end of the hour, he was thoroughly spent—yet invigorated. He said he felt two inches taller. His back felt looser. Better yet, he was ready to try it again the next day.

From that day forward, Dallas did yoga workouts. I am extremely proud of Page for picking up yoga, and amazed that his ego-integrity would allow him to celebrate his maleness through the practice. I have no doubt that he will build an army of shirtless, sweaty, smiling yogis doing his brand of YRG—and that's a sight a girl can appreciate!

THE OWNER'S MANUAL

HOW TO USE THIS BOOK

If you're a Regular Guy like me, I'm sure you would never read an owner's manual for anything you buy, even when it means learning about safety or perhaps a better understanding of the new tool, gadget, or toy you just bought. But this section will help you get the most out of this book, so suck it up and read this, men!

First, in Chapter 1, you'll learn all you need to know to prepare you for your Yoga for Regular Guys workout. You will learn the *hows* and *whys* of breathing properly. If you're thinking, "What, I'm breathin', what else do you need?" well, then you must check out the breathing technique section (p. 18). We'll also give you the background information about your maximum aerobic function/target heart rate: what it is, how it works, and how to find your own optimal target rate. Remember, I promised to keep it stupidly simple. You will understand why you need a heart rate monitor and how to get the most out of your workouts.

The "Yoga for Regular Guys" workout in Chapter 2 gives you the goods. You get pictures, descriptions, and everything else you need to get started on the program that can change your life. We break up the 20-minute yoga workout into sections to help you learn more quickly and have a foundation to build on when working up to a 30- or 45-minute workout.

In "Hammers and Duct Tape," Chapter 3, you will learn some quick fixes for instant stress relief, along with some incredible therapy and rehab techniques that I have used over the years for my bad knees, shoulders, hips, and back. No, I'm not talking about sex for stress relief—not that there's anything wrong with that. But we will show you how to do a few simple exercises that could lower your stress levels *and* help your joints, in a lot less time than it would take to find some sex. Plus, unlike sex release, our stress relief exercises can be done anywhere, anytime. We even added some exercises that will help you increase your heart rate and strengthen your core. Use the "Hammers and Duct Tape" chapter upon waking, before bed, or any time you need a quick fix.

In Chapter 4, "DDP's Health Tips and Preventative Maintenance," we will clue you in to some of the best health secrets I learned from the Yoga-Doc, along with road-tested regimens, such as organic juicing, using ice and heat, applied kinesiology and massage, keeping hydrated, and a no-nonsense way to eat that can transform you into a lean, mean fightin' machine.

The final chapter gives you the inspiration and motivation to put down the TV remote and get ready to *heat up, get healthy, and stay hard*!

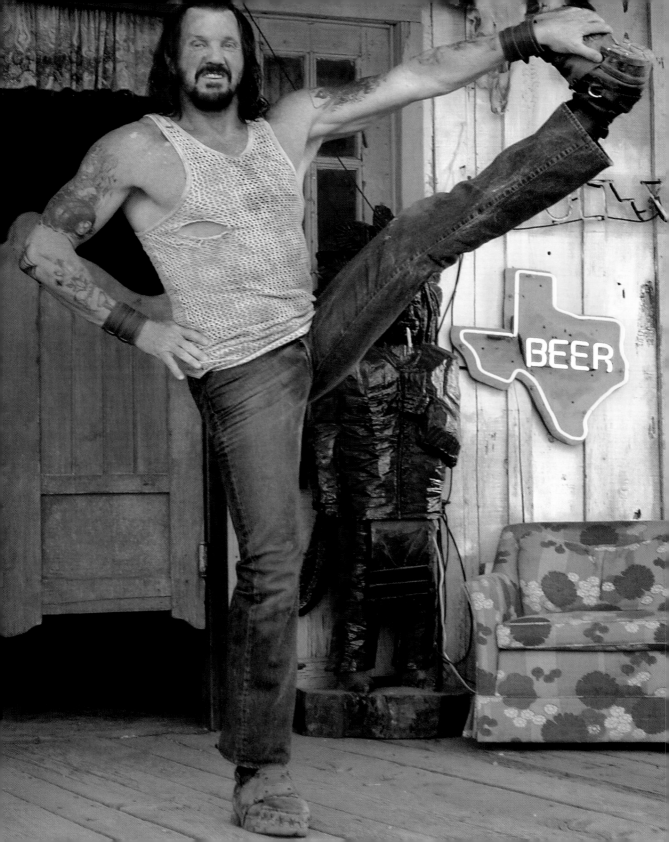

CHAPTER 1

GETTING READY FOR YRG

Believe it or not, *breathing* is the most important part of YRG. Why? Because when you are breathing properly, you will find that you can go deeper into your yoga positions, which will increase your flexibility and raise your heart rate. And what's the best way to measure your heart rate? By wearing a *heart monitor*. Let's face it: Guys love stats. You want to know how much you can bench press. You want to know how fast you can run (or used to run). You want to see your results right before your eyes, and you want to see them immediately. But, the main reason you wear a heart monitor is to keep your heart rate in the optimal cardio and fat-burning zones to get the most out of your YRG workout. If you're breathing fully while staying in your cardio/fat-burning zone for the entire YRG workout, you'll be kickin' ass and takin' names in no time!

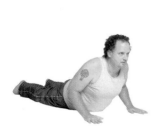

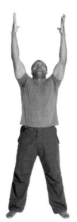

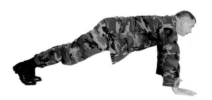

◄ This is me as Billy Ray Snapper from *Devil's Rejects*, doing a not-so-regular YRG position. Don't worry—I'm not going to make you do this. —DDP

YA GOTTA BELIEVE, IT'S ALL ABOUT HOW YOU BREATHE!

This section focuses on proper breathing techniques not only when doing Yoga for Regular Guys, but also when you need to calm down, focus, and de-stress. Hundreds of books have been written on the subject. In this book we will touch on the importance of the breath while doing yoga.

If you're not breathing correctly or not breathing at all while doing yoga, all you're doing is stretching, and according to many experts, stretching will only get you so far. But when you stretch and move in concert with your breath, you are doing yoga, which is a total body exercise. And when you're doing yoga properly, you're gaining physical and mental focus, balance, endurance, flexibility, and power. How important is breathing to us? Remember, you can go without food for weeks. You can go without water for days. But if you go without oxygen for more than a few minutes, it's curtains—sudden death without the overtime—fade to black.

It All Starts with Your First Breath

YOGA-DOC SAYS . . .

At birth, the first thing the doctor does is to check the many aspects of a newborn child's respiration with an "APGAR" score that measures the baby's heart rate, respiratory effort, muscle tone, response to stimuli, and skin color. These five indicators all relate to a newborn's ability to breathe and properly utilize oxygen. The old saying goes, you know that your newborn is healthy if it comes out kicking and screaming.

As Regular Guys, we also know that the reason we came out kicking and screaming is because at the time of birth, we knew that we just left a warm, soft, and wonderful place that we were going to spend a major part of our lives trying to hump, dive, or climb back into! (Now I don't care who you are, that was some funny shit right there.)

Healthy babies breathe into their whole lung fields, from the belly to the collarbones. When we breathe this way in our yoga workouts, we get clean, oxygenated blood to places in our body that we didn't even know we had. Deep, long, slow breathing in concert with yoga movements stretches and rejuvenates the body from the inside to the outside. This type of breathing and moving also helps create space between each vertebra and assists in healing compressed spinal discs; it squeezes tired/trapped blood out of our vital organs and brings fresh oxygenated blood back to those same organs. It also helps break up old scar tissue and fix our posture.

Why We Slouch on the Couch

Unfortunately, as we accumulate physical traumas in our lives, such as sports injuries, car accidents, pile drivers/tombstones, falls, or even steel chairs to the skull, an accumulation of scar tissue forms around those old injuries. These traumas create structural "holding patterns" in our body, which cause loss of flexibility as well as distortions in our posture. Even smaller traumas, such as slouching on the couch, sleeping on airplanes, long periods of inactivity, driving for long hours, or sitting for hours at the computer can create bad postural habits. According to the Yoga-Doc, in time, these "postural distortions" and regions of accumulated stress will cause our body to close down and fold inward, which leads to decreased lung capacity—which could cause the depth of our breath to become shallower and shallower. Shallow breathing means less efficient blood-oxygen exchange and could lead to a lot of physical problems.

How Can Yoga Help?

You may ask, "Can yoga help change or prevent all of this?" The answer is, YES! Regular yoga workouts can assist in loosening you up and straightening you out!

The Yoga-Doc taught me a lot about how yoga helps the brain and nervous system. So now I'll break it all down into a language that I call "Regular Guy-ese." When we take deep, long, slow breaths, we can actually stop the "fight or flight" portion of our nervous system (called the sympathetic nervous system) from overreacting to different types of stress. The sympathetic nervous system goes into high gear when our brain activates it in the presence of perceived danger. We absolutely need the sympathetic system when we are in physical danger because it prepares our body to either do some serious ass whoopin' or run like hell if necessary. It is a lot like having a nitrous oxide tank hooked up to your hot rod. You know that you should use it only when you absolutely need it, because if you fire it up too often, it will tear apart the inner workings of your vehicle.

Unfortunately, our brain fires up our sympathetic system even when it is inappropriate to physically run or fight, such as during heavy-duty emotional situations or confrontational work issues. It might be inappropriate to kick your boss's ass while he or she is attempting to verbally rip you a new one. When your body goes into this stress response, you have all this serious go-go juice coursing through your system, including adrenalin and cortisol, with no place to burn it off. It's like firing up your nitrous oxide tank and slamming on the brakes at the same time. Talk about tearing yourself up inside!

When people see you reacting to stress, they tell you to take some deep breaths to calm down. Of course, when you are in the middle of something hot, you may not see the benefits of taking a few deep, slow breaths. You may even want to "choke-out" (as wrestlers say) the person who was trying to mellow you out. However, a few deep, slow breaths, preferably through the nostrils, can slow down the sympathetic system's fight or flight response. Those deep, slow breaths can also activate what's known as the parasympathetic nervous system. The parasympathetic nervous system is responsible for sleep, digestion, reproduction, and the healing response. I like to call it the breed, feed, and Z's system. We definitely need a whole lot more of that.

YOGA-DOC SAYS . . .

It is extremely important to be very conscious of how you breathe while doing your Yoga for Regular Guys program. Deep, long, slow breaths through your nose, taken in concert with each movement, can maximize your benefits tenfold! Breathing through the nostrils gives you more rib and lung expansion for a longer period of time, thereby optimizing the oxygenation process and increasing blood flow.

If you follow my cues, you will be doing some serious exercise, losing weight, and getting in great shape while still flowing in the parasympathetic zone. This program emphasizes exercising in a state of calm, focused movement and breathing without the fight or flight response. And remember, this is not competitive yoga! If you want to compete with someone or something, compete with yourself by seeing how long you can perform this kick-ass workout while staying calm and breathing deeply.

How to Breathe While Doing the YRG Workout

Do you remember when I promised that I would keep things stupidly simple?

The breathing technique for your YRG workout may appear ridiculously easy to perform, because all I'm asking you to do is breathe slowly and deeply through your nostrils, a.k.a. your nose holes, for the entire program. If you try to consciously fill your entire body with oxygen each time I ask you to inhale, you will break up the tension that lives in the different corners of your body. You will get even greater benefits if you try to "push" each inhalation into those tight spots. Exhale in a slow and controlled manner through your nose, and only through your nose if possible. Bring tissues, a towel, or use your sleeve if you have to, but I'm tellin' ya, this workout might knock the snot right out of you!

Now, the ridiculously tough part about this breathing technique is that I'm asking you to completely focus on each and every breath you take for the entire 20, 30, or 45 minutes. Just remember, you have to do this focused type of breathing while you are stretching, squatting, twisting, or trying to hold a position that makes you feel as if your legs or arms have caught fire! I am absolutely certain that you will completely blank out on your breathing focus at least a thousand times while you learn these workouts. (I can't begin to tell you how tough it was for me to get the breathing down.) So don't be discouraged if you are having a hard time with the coordinated breathing at first.

All you have to do is follow my cadence and **focus, focus, focus**. I will let you know when to inhale and exhale. Hang in there!

The breathing exercise below helps you calm your mind and relax your body in a minute or less! When you breathe this way, you enable your body to fully utilize every bit of oxygen that you take in and pump it directly into your bloodstream for immediate use. Plus, you are expelling carbon dioxide (CO_2) and other waste products very efficiently on each exhalation.

"But I *Do* Breathe Properly!" . . . No, I'll Bet You Don't!

Trust me, it's going to take practice to learn to breathe properly. If you read the foreword by Rob Zombie (which is funny as hell . . . thanks RZ), you know he *thought* he knew how to breathe—but he didn't. Most people don't, aside from Olympic swimmers and opera singers. I now know how to breathe properly, but it took me three months before I didn't have to think about it anymore. Once my breathing became automatic, my flexibility improved by leaps and bounds.

If you watch a baby breathe, you will see his or her stomach expand with each inhalation and contract with each exhalation. We all breathe properly when we are born, but before you know it, stress creeps into our lives and changes everything. So, here's the KISS breathing technique:

1. Sit in a comfortable position on a chair or on the floor, lie on your back, or just stand in an upright position.
2. Inhale through your nose gently and deeply. Slowly fill your lungs, then your stomach, full of air. That's right: your stomach, your belly, and your gut push out like Santa Claus as you pull all that air deeply into your lungs and then your stomach. Yes, I said your stomach!
3. Once you have filled your stomach full of air, slowly exhale through your nose, controlling that exhalation until every last bit of CO_2 leaves you. As you do this, pull your stomach in toward your rib cage; that's right, bucko—suck in your stomach as you are pushing out the air.
4. Now inhale once again. Repeat the cycle five more times, and feel the buzz!

I know it's not going to feel natural for you to be breathing through your stomach, but you have to trust me. It will continually help you get deeper into each of your positions day by day. Repeat this exercise daily and you will own it.

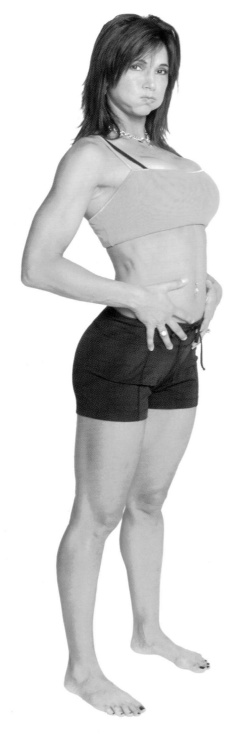

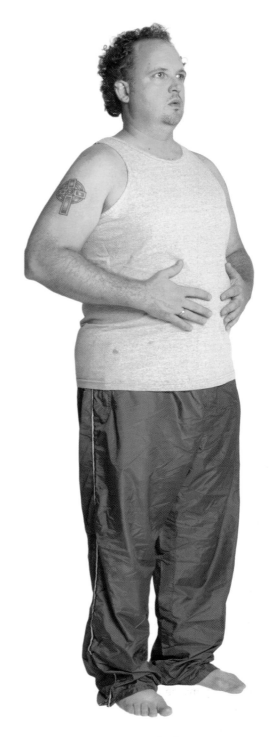

inhale

exhale

YA GOTTA HAVE HEART

Okay guys, it's time to get your heart on! Yes, yoga can help you get a healthier heart without punishing your knees in the process. You'll actually be *strengthening* your knees and maximizing your aerobic heart rate by wearing a heart monitor.

The Formula to Success: Get Your Heart On

Let me tell you why I wear a heart monitor. The main man responsible for keeping DDP in the ring all of these years is a guy named Dr. Ken West, an applied kinesiologist. One day, Doc West was working on me—the usual two-hour session. And he was telling me about Mark Allen: Mark had won the Hawaii Triathlon three years in a row, but his streak came to an end when he turned thirty-five. He was going to retire, when he heard about the heart monitor work that his kinesiologist, Dr. Phil Maffetone, had been working on.

Dr. Maffetone believes you can get the most out of your body by controlling your heart rate using a basic formula: Let's say you're forty years old. Subtract 40 from 180, which gives you 140. If you keep your heart rate between 120 and 140 beats per minute (bpms), you will burn fat and increase your stamina. Now if you're an athlete, you can take that 140 up to 145 bpms, and if you are an *extreme* athlete, push it up to 150 bpms, but not for long periods of time. (Like a hot rod, you don't want to bury the needle in the red zone for long, or something's gonna blow.)

The bottom line is that Mark followed these instructions, and the next thing you know, he wins the Ironman again when he's thirty-six, thirty-seven, and thirty-eight years old before deciding to retire. That's pretty amazing, considering that the Hawaii Ironman is the mack daddy of all triathlons. They run twenty-six miles, swim five miles, then get on a bike and ride 150 miles—good Gawd!

I wanted to incorporate that formula into my workout, so I started wearing my heart monitor on the StairMaster and in the gym while I was lifting weights. One day I even wore it to a power yoga class. I wasn't really paying attention to the monitor while I was working out. But about two-thirds of the way through the class, I glanced at my monitor, and I was amazed that my heart rate was at 152 bpms. I was doing Warrior Two; I thought to myself, wow, this is a great angle to prove to the Regular Guy that this stuff works. (The whole yoga-babes angle came much later.)

I love having my heart monitor on because it helps me push myself, and it also lets me know when to back off. In this section, we're going to talk about the importance of maintaining your maximum aerobic heart rate while exercising. We're going to start by learning the difference between glycogen-burning anaerobic exercise and continuous fat-burning/cardiovascular exercise.

Put very simply, when you are walking, running, biking, cross-country skiing, doing yoga, or having sex for 20 or 60 minutes while operating at your maximum aerobic heart rate or 20 to 25 bpm less, you are performing *cardiovascular exercise*. You're utilizing your aerobic energy system, which burns fat as its fuel source.

If you are engaging in any competitive sport that pushes your heart rate past your target maximum aerobic heart rate for prolonged periods of time, whether you're sprinting, slam dancing, or weightlifting, you are performing *anaerobic exercise*. Anaerobic exercise is much less efficient, burns sugar as its fuel source, and utilizes the lactic acid energy pathway, requiring more recovery time.

Let's face it, guys, many of us have enough fat stores to keep our aerobic system going for a long time, so we better get started soon!

Don't Redline Your Hot Rod

I said earlier that your body functions a lot like a car. When you are out driving, your car has a certain level of rpms and a specific range of speed where it operates with maximum fuel efficiency and minimal wear and tear on its parts.

YOGA DOC SAYS . . .

When we exercise, our aerobic system, heart, lungs, and entire circulatory system operate at the most energy-efficient level, known as the Maximum Aerobic Function. Dr. Philip Maffetone's book, *In Fitness and in Health*, defines the Maximum Aerobic Function as the maximum level of exercise that an individual can perform while utilizing his or her aerobic, fat-burning energy system. In short, it is the most exercise your body can perform using the highly efficient, fat-burning aerobic system just before it downshifts into the less efficient, sugar-burning, anaerobic, lactic acid energy pathway. And the best tool you can use to indicate whether you are utilizing your aerobic system during exercise is the heart rate monitor.

Using a heart rate monitor will help keep your body at the optimal fat-burning zone/target heart rate. Using the formula developed by Dr. Maffetone and six-time Ironman Champion Mark Allen, you can easily customize your target/maximum aerobic heart rate to your specific situation. Here it is again, spelled out a little differently, so you can tailor it to your own needs:

- If you have been exercising regularly for two years or less, or if you have been exercising for a longer period but not as regularly, your target heart rate is 180 beats per minute minus your age.
- If you are overcoming a major illness or taking regular medication, you should subtract

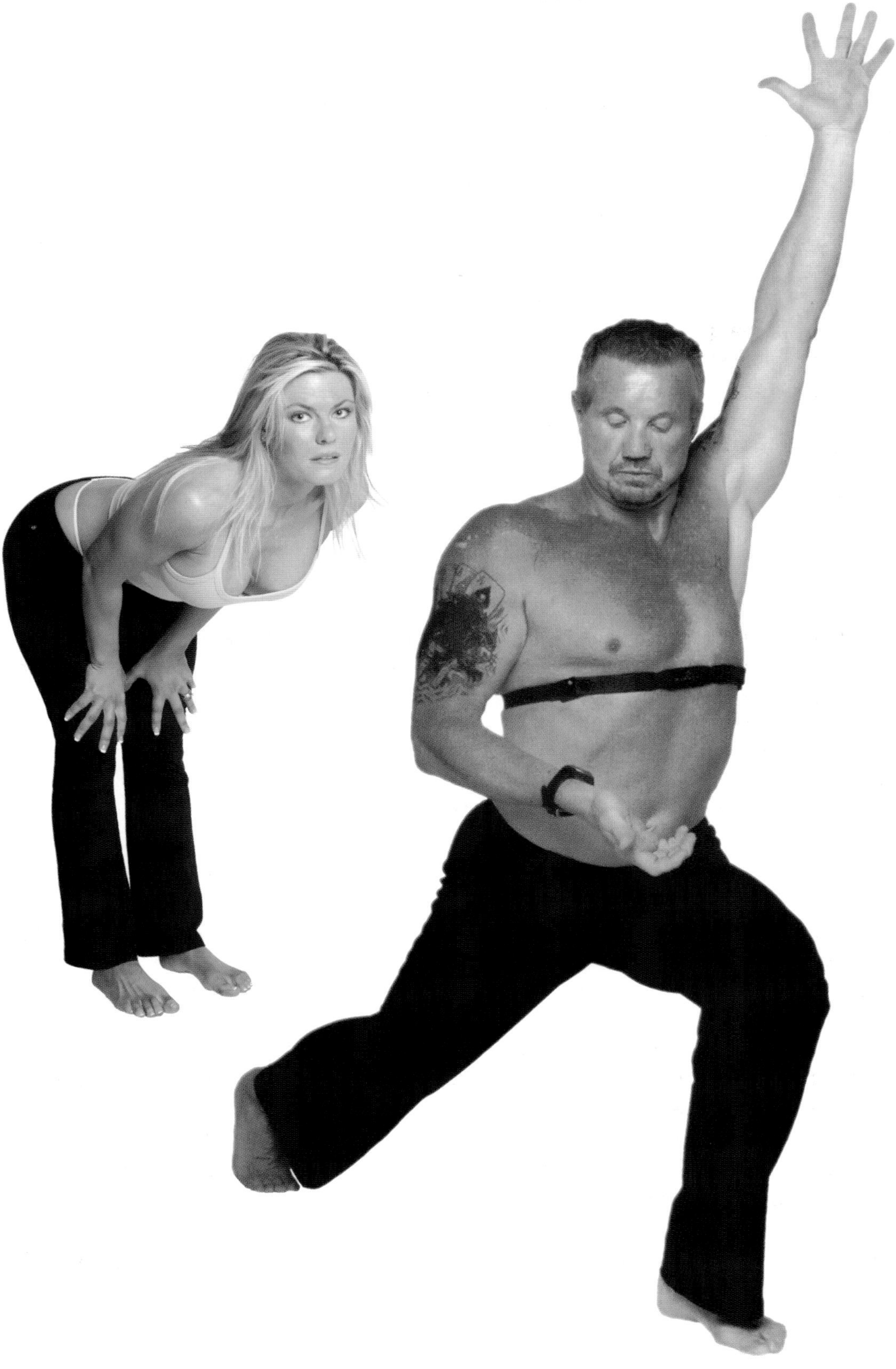

an additional ten beats per minute from your original target heart rate.

- If you tend to catch colds easily or if you are not currently exercising, whether by choice or due to injury, you should subtract five beats per minute from your original target heart rate.
- If you have been exercising regularly for more than two years without injury, add five to ten beats per minute to your target heart rate.

Now that you understand how your target heart rate works, you are ready to purchase your heart monitor and start the Yoga for Regular Guys workout.

Strap One On

Most heart monitors have the same working parts. Just purchase the most basic heart monitor you can find. You have a strap or receiver that wraps around your lower ribcage, just below your nipples. This part actually tracks each beat of your heart. You also have the wristwatch portion, known as the monitor, which displays how many times your heart beats per minute. To set up your heart monitor, just follow the simple instructions that come with it and you'll be all set! It's way easier than setting up your TiVo.

The Yoga for Regular Guys workout is designed like all great exercise programs. It starts you out with an easy **warm-up** of approximately 5 to 7 minutes to get your blood flowing and your joints warm. Your heart rate will steadily rise throughout the warm-up.

The **working phase** of the YRG workout is anywhere from 10 to 31 minutes in duration, depending upon which YRG workout you are doing. This is the hardest part of the workout and requires you to hold positions that engage your entire body. This is where you should be near your maximum aerobic heart rate or only as low as 25 bpms below your max. If you can sustain your heart rate within this range for the working phase of the YRG workout, you'll be burning fat while getting fit, flexible, and focused.

The **cool-down** phase takes about 5 to 7 minutes, and it is designed to stretch you out and bring your heart rate back down slowly.

YOGA DOC SAYS . . .

Remember, it's okay to be 20 to 25 beats below your maximum aerobic heart rate while doing this program; you will still burn fat, though at a slightly lower rate. It's also okay if your heart rate spikes above your max for a few seconds, but it is very important to stay at or below your maximum rate to stay out of the anaerobic, glycogen-burning zone. When exercise hits the anaerobic zone, it should only be for a short time; otherwise, it could put undue stress on your body and put you into the fight or flight, sympathetic nervous system response—*not* a good thing.

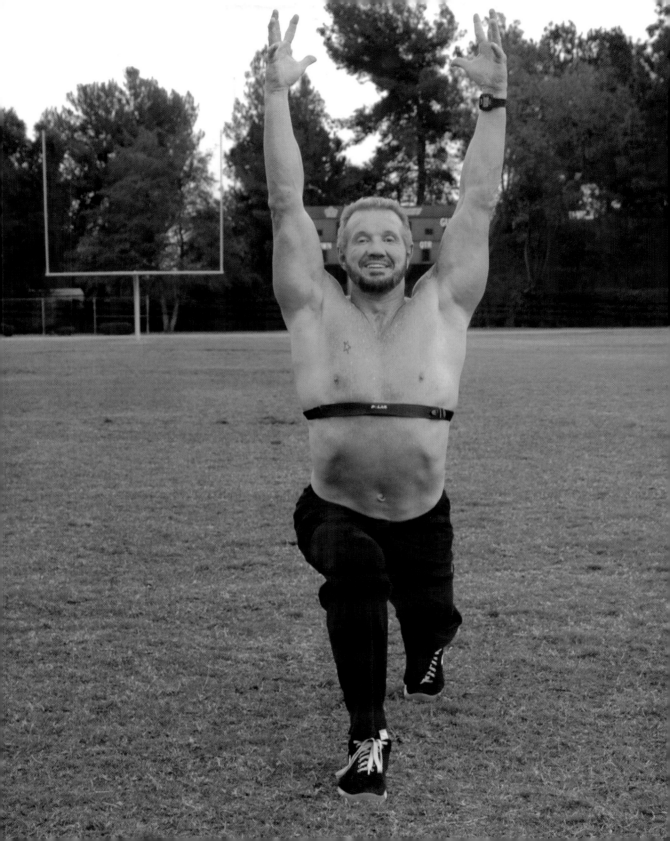

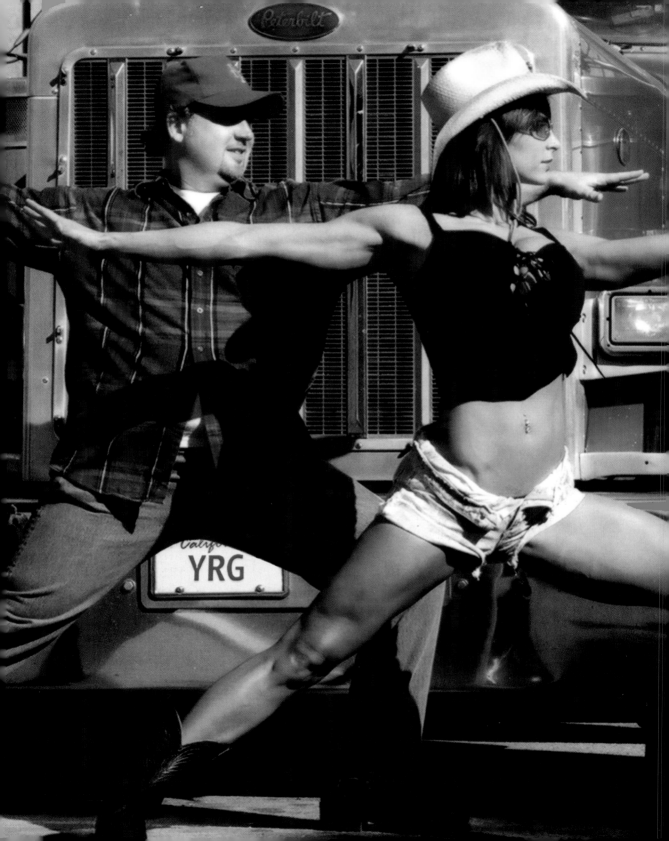

CHAPTER 2

PUTTING IT ALL TOGETHER

This chapter is where it all comes together! Follow the Regular Guys and yoga-babes (good Gawd!) as they lead the way through this mack daddy workout that will help you tune up, get flexible, and stay hard. The workout is broken into sections so that you always have a goal to work toward. Check out the **Diamond Cutter**, my patented wrestling finishing move: it shows up at the end of almost every section to put the BANG into your workout and to remind you that you *did* it!

You are now on your way to learning what you need to start a healthier and more fulfilling lifestyle. Remember to work at your own pace—this isn't competitive yoga. Just keep at it and anything is possible. Now get to work!

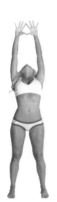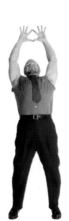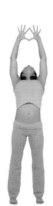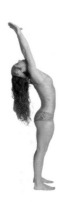

20 ›MINUTE WORKOUT SECTIONS

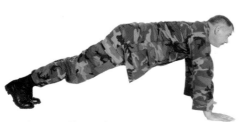

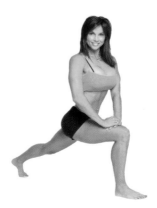

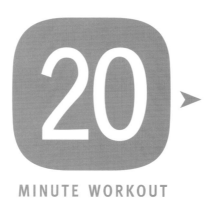

MINUTE WORKOUT

The 20-Minute Workout is the platform on which all the other workouts are based. So this is the most important YRG workout for you to learn.

The main reason I came up with the 20-Minute Workout is because people were always telling me: "DDP, I'd love to do your YRG workout, but I just don't have the time." My response is always the same: "Do you have twenty minutes?" And they say, "Well, of course I've got twenty minutes." Then I would say, "Well, you've got the time—that's all you need to start to change your life, bro." As I say throughout this book, *flexibility is youth*, and if you spend two to three days a week doing this 20-Minute Workout, I'm telling you, your flexibility will start to come back. Trust me, you will feel younger, and isn't that what everyone wants to feel—younger?

Just twenty minutes a day will start to loosen up your joints and your muscles. It will help you avoid injury, and you can have a healthier, happier sex life. I know I've got you on the sex life deal—but it's true. So read this twenty-minute section a couple of times, and get to know the program, and of course check out the hot yoga-babes. Then put the book on the floor next to you for reference. Roll out your yoga mat, and let's do it!

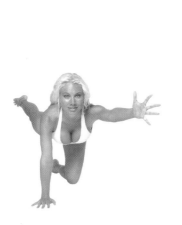

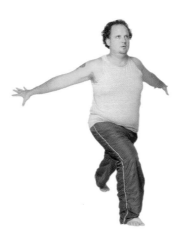

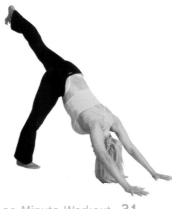

◄ IGNITION

Okay guys, this is where it all begins. Ignition is that time during a rocket launch countdown where the ship is just about ready to lift off!

This initial section of the YRG workout is about knocking the rust off. It's designed to make you tune into your breathing while performing very simple stretches and movements in a slow and easy manner. It's a lot like checking your hot rod's air intake and exhaust systems, gear shifter, and brakes just before you fire it up and let 'er rip!

The **Deep Belly Breathing** gives you all the fuel/energy you need to keep that oxygen flowing steadily throughout your workout. Plus, we set the tone for the entire YRG workout by connecting to our breathing from the very beginning while allowing the continuous and constant flow of breath to get you through your workouts when the seas get rough and you're feeling lost.

So focus on your Deep Belly Breathing while we fire it up and *get this party started!*

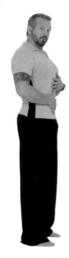

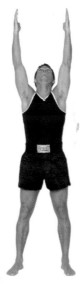

3

DEEP BELLY BREATHING—EXHALE
Then slowly exhale out of your nostrils, and let your body push all of the air out of your body while sucking your stomach to the back of your spine. Your hands are in position so you can feel your body expand with each inhalation and contract with each exhalation. Yes, pull your stomach back to your spine. Take three deep breaths.

4

TOUCHDOWN
Inhale and reach your arms into a touchdown signal. Roll your shoulders back while keeping your palms facing each other and look up at your hands.

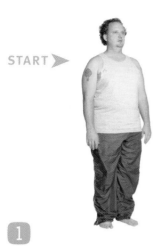

1

MOUNTAIN POSITION

Standing tall, step your feet hip-width apart. Now spread your toes wide, straighten your legs, and gently suck that big, beautiful belly inward. Lift your chest, and roll your shoulders back. Make sure that your head is in line with your shoulders. This is your perfect standing position. In this position, you're not just any mountain, you're Mount Freakin' Everest!

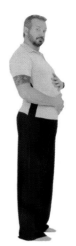

► **2**

DEEP BELLY BREATHING—INHALE

Gentlemen, start your engines by putting the palm of your right hand on your belly button and your left hand just above it. Now breathe deeply through your nostrils and fill your belly up, pushing your stomach out like Santa Claus, then fill your solar plexus, and finally your entire chest with pure oxygen. Push that stomach out!

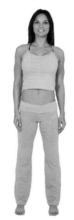

► **5**

MOUNTAIN POSITION

Exhale as you slowly lower your arms back down to your sides. Repeat Touchdown to Mountain Position two more times as we begin to blast air into the furnace.

HOT TIP!

It doesn't matter whether you are sporting six-pack abs or if you're carrying a beer keg under your shirt—if you are breathing correctly, you'll feel each breath energize your body while your mind gets focused like a laser.

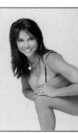

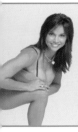

FIRE UP THE BACK AND THE HIPS

As we continue to warm up, this sequence stretches your back, hamstrings, and Achilles tendons. It also strengthens the quads and lower back, along with all of the muscles that surround the hips and knees. As you move through this sequence, I guarantee that you will begin to *feel the fire!*

This may be the one sequence I do every day of my life. Actually, I end up doing it a couple of times a day when I'm running hard. This exercise can be used to warm up before running, playing tennis, golfing, or just getting ready for work. It strengthens the low back along with all of the muscles that surround the hips and knees. If you're ever on a long flight with me, and you happen to be sitting in first class, you will most likely see me doing this in the front of the plane—and, no, I'm not bullshitting you.

HOT TIP!

As you continue through this workout, you will see that everyone does the position a little differently. If you need to bend your knees to be comfortable in a certain position, or if you can't do a position at all, it's okay. Take your time. It's the groovin' of the smoothin'. And if you go to a yoga class, take a tip from DDP and never pick the front row—go for the middle. That way you can focus on yoga-babes in all directions.

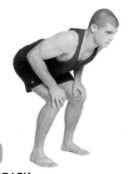

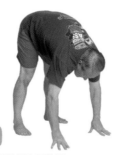

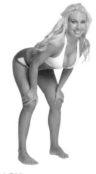

3

BARBACK
Inhale and slide your hands up to your knees. Lift your head, roll your shoulders back, slide your heels out a bit, and feel your hips open up. If you have to, you can bend your knees.

4

FORWARD BEND
Exhale and fold forward while sliding your hands back down your shins and to the floor, if you can manage it. Repeat Barback to Forward Bend two more times.

5

BARBACK
Come back into Barback as you inhale, bending your knees a bit if you have to. Slide your hands up to your knees, lift your head, roll your shoulders back, and slide your heels out a bit.

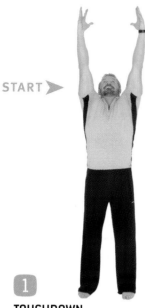

1
TOUCHDOWN
Inhale and reach up
into a Touchdown signal.

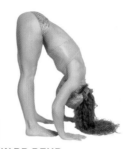

2
FORWARD BEND
Exhale, and hinge forward at the hips as
you slide your hands down your shins.
Hang for five deep inhalations and exhalations.

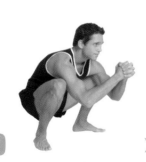

6
CATCHER'S POSITION
Exhale and sink into Catcher's
Position by bending your knees
and slowly squatting like the great
Yogi Berra. Squat as deeply as you
can as you lift your torso and try
to get your heels flat on the floor.
Sit for three deep breaths.

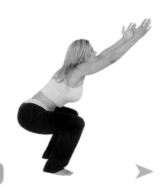

7
REACH AND RISE
Inhale and reach your arms to
the sky with palms facing each
other while you squeeze your
knees a little closer.

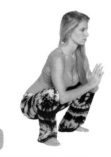

8
CATCHER'S POSITION
Exhale, and sink deeper into
Catcher's Position. Repeat
Catcher's Position to Reach and
Rise two more times.

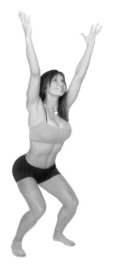

9 THUNDERBOLT

Inhale, lift your ass off the ground, and raise your chest and hips a little. Reach your arms toward the sky, and with each inhalation, try reaching a little higher.

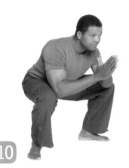

10 CATCHER'S POSITION

Now squat and drop back into Catcher's Position. Repeat Thunderbolt to Catcher's Position two more times.

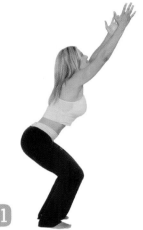

11 THUNDERBOLT

Come into Thunderbolt once again. Inhale, lift your ass off the ground, and raise your chest and hips a little as you reach your arms toward the sky.

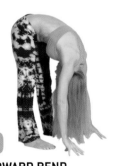

12 FORWARD BEND

Exhale, straighten your legs, and hang for one deep breath.

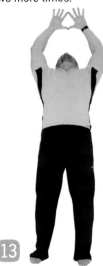

13 DIAMOND CUTTER

Inhale, take a deep breath, and roll up one vertebra at a time. Tighten your belly, and reach your arms up to the sky, making the Diamond Cutter Sign while arching back.

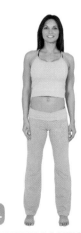

14 MOUNTAIN POSITION

Exhale and feel the BANG as you lower your arms back down to your sides.

TOUCHDOWNS AND SIDE BENDS

This section will open your shoulders, activate your core stabilizing muscles (which surround your abdomen and lumbar spine) *and* make you as tall as you're supposed to be. You might ask, "Make me as tall as I'm supposed to be—what, am I shrinking or something?"

Well, have you ever felt so compressed and smooshed after a long day that you thought your ass was sitting up on your shoulders? I know I sure have!

In fact, according to the Yoga-Doc, our discs *do* compress and we *do* shrink some after a long day of standing, desk work, or driving.

So focus on keeping your head in line with your spine during this sequence as you put a little more space between your ass and your neck.

START ▶

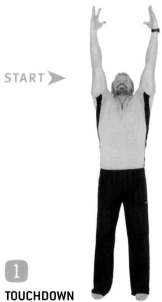

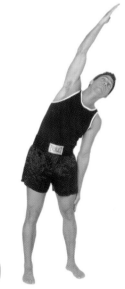

1

TOUCHDOWN
Inhale with feet at hips' width. Reach your arms into a Touchdown signal, roll your shoulders back while keeping your palms facing each other, and look up at your hands.

2

SIDE BEND RIGHT
Exhale as you drop your left hand to your side. Now inhale as you reach your right hand skyward, and look up at that hand as you squeeze your belly toward your spine. Exhale and slide your left hand down your side while rolling your right shoulder back. Take three deep breaths here.

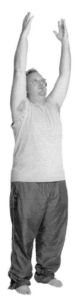

3

TOUCHDOWN

Now inhale back up into Touchdown, and roll your shoulders back while keeping your palms facing each other, and look up at your hands.

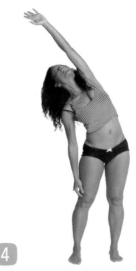

4

SIDE BEND LEFT

Exhale as you drop your right hand to your side. Now inhale and reach your left hand skyward, and look up at that hand as you squeeze your belly toward your spine. Exhale and slide your right hand down your side while rolling your left shoulder back. Take three deep breaths here.

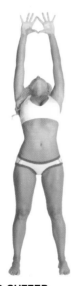

5

DIAMOND CUTTER

Inhale, tighten your belly, and reach both arms to the sky. Make the Diamond Cutter Sign while arching back.

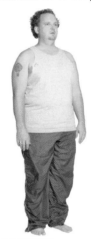

6

MOUNTAIN POSITION

Exhale, and lower your hands down to your sides into Mountain Position.

RAINING CATS, DOGS, AND COBRAS

This is a great sequence that flexes, extends, and stabilizes the muscles that surround your spine. **Cat Lifts** and **Cat Arches** knock out the kinks. **Cobra** is one of the great quick fixes for all you guys who spend way too much time driving or hunched over a computer screen. **Down Dog** is the best all-in-one position that opens your chest, shoulders, neck, low back, hamstrings, and calves.

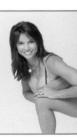

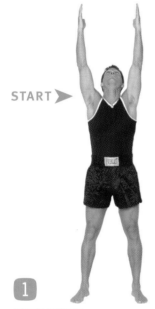

START ➤

HOT TIP!
This is your one-stop shop for destroying bad postural habits, which fold you inward and decrease your lung capacity. Don't forget to breathe while you do this. You know what they say about guys with small lungs …

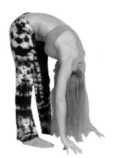

1

TOUCHDOWN
Inhale and reach up into a Touchdown signal.

➤ **2**

FORWARD BEND
Exhale, reach out, and fold forward.

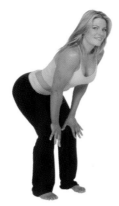

3
BARBACK

Inhale, bend your knees a bit, and slide your hands up to your knees. Lift your head and roll your shoulders back as you slide your heels out a bit and feel your hips open up.

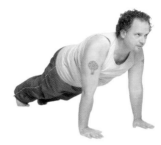

4
PUSH-UP POSITION

Exhale, lower your hands to the mat, and step or jump back into a push-up position.

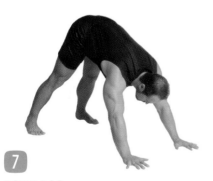

7
DOWN DOG

Exhale and push back into Down Dog by lifting your hips while you straighten your arms and press your chest back toward your legs. Relax your neck, straighten your legs, and press your heels down. If your heels are nowhere near the floor, don't worry about it. This takes time. Take three deep breaths.

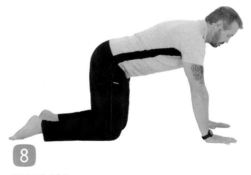

8
TABLE TOP

Drop to your knees and press your hands into the floor directly below your shoulders.

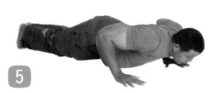

5

LOWER DOWN

Lower your body down slowly 3 . . . 2 . . . 1, until you are three inches off the ground while squeezing your elbows in toward your ribs and making sure that your shoulders don't dip below your elbows. Now, hold and hover over your mat, if possible, for a count 3 . . . 2 . . . 1. Then fully exhale and lower yourself to the ground.

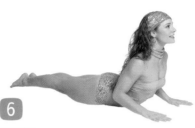

6

COBRA

Inhale and lengthen into Cobra with your hands pressing into the floor and your elbows in close to your ribs. Now lift your chest up and roll your shoulders back like a king cobra snake. Keep the tops of your feet, the fronts of your legs, and your pelvis pressed gently into the floor. Now pick a point to focus on. It may be the hot looking yoga-babe in front of you. Take three deep breaths.

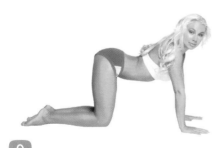

9

CAT LIFT

Inhale, lift your head, roll your shoulders back, and let your belly relax.

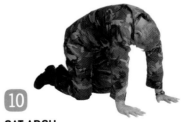

10

CAT ARCH

Exhale and look back at your beltline as you arch up like an angry cat. Take two more reps of Cat Lift to Cat Arch.

BROKEN TABLE

Effective spinal rehab needs the following components: strengthening, stretching, balance, and traction. This exercise sequence has it all. We also introduce the **Child's Position**, which is the tired guy's version of Down Dog. Drop into Child's Position any time you need a breather.

HOT TIP!
This exercise sequence not only strengthens your core, it also helps get you that tight ass you have always wanted. (On your own backside, not in your hand!) Look no further than each of the yoga-babes for the perfect specimen.

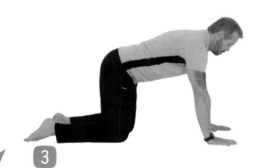

3

TABLE TOP
Exhale and move back into Table Top.

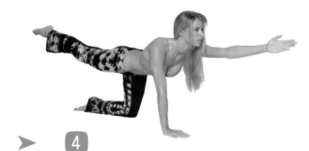

4

LEFT TABLE TOP TRACTION
Inhale as you move to the opposite side. Lift and push your right leg straight back while you strongly reach your left arm straight ahead. Take three deep breaths.

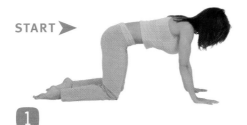

1

TABLE TOP
Inhale and move to Table Top.

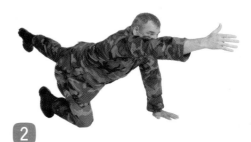

>

2

RIGHT TABLE TOP TRACTION
Raise your left leg straight back with intention while reaching your right arm straight ahead as if stretching out to shake someone's hand. Take three deep breaths while you engage your arm muscles and leg muscles strongly.

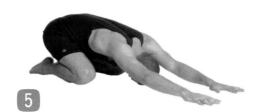

>

5

CHILD'S POSITION
Exhale and push your ass back toward your heels while reaching your arms far forward and resting your forehead on the ground. This is Child's Position. Take three deep breaths.

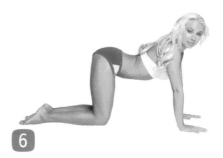

>

6

CAT LIFT
Inhale and return to Cat Lift.

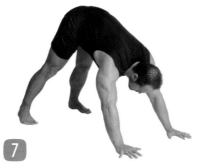

7

DOWN DOG

Exhale, curl your toes under, push your hips up, and straighten your arms as you press into Down Dog. Take one deep inhalation.

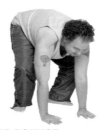

8

LEAP AND POUNCE

Exhale as you step or jump with both of your feet right behind your hands, keeping your knees bent.

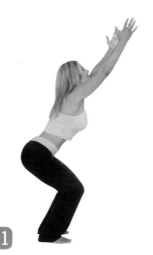

11

THUNDERBOLT

Inhale, and lift your ass, chest, shoulders, and arms skyward while you squeeze your knees a little closer. Now look up at your hands. Pretend that you're sitting on a chair.

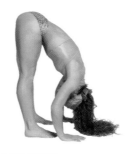

12

FORWARD BEND

Exhale, straighten your legs, and hang forward.

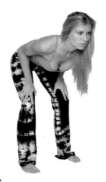

9

BARBACK
Inhale, slide your hands up to your knees, flatten your back, and press your heels out slightly.

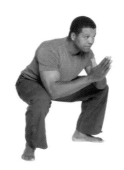

10

CATCHER'S POSITION
Exhale, drop, and squat. See if you can keep your heels flat on the floor.

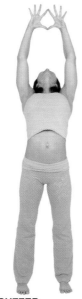

13

DIAMOND CUTTER
Inhale, reach both arms up into the Diamond Cutter Sign, and lean way back.

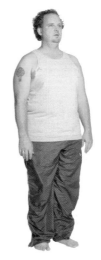

14

MOUNTAIN POSITION
Exhale and feel the BANG as you lower your arms back down to your sides.

GET HOT
DDP's Modified Sun Salutation for Guys

Now it's time to turn it up and burn. This section is designed to bump up your heart-rate toward your maximum aerobic number. We have taken yoga's traditional **Sun Salutations**, of which there are three types, and melted them all down into one. **Barback**, which is a good back and hip stabilizer, and **Catcher's Position** have been added to allow for more back and hip flexibility while moving through this sequence. We also modified the opening stance from "knees together" to a more useful, athletic, and less ball-crushing "hip-width" stance. (You're welcome, guys.) We found that the slightly wider stance helps activate the muscles of the entire thigh throughout this section of the YRG workout. We also added the **Diamond Cutter** to the Sun Salutation to reset your posture and put *the Bang* into this great warm-up.

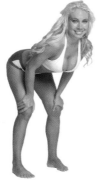

3 BARBACK
Inhale, bend your knees, slide your hands up to your knees, and lift your head as you roll your shoulders back. Slide your heels out a bit and feel your hips open.

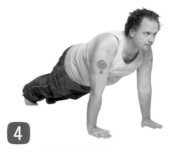

4 PUSH-UP POSITION
Lower your hands to the mat, and step or jump back into a push-up position.

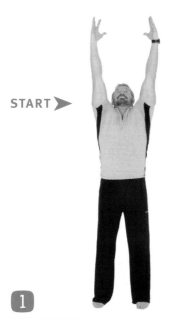

1
TOUCHDOWN
Inhale and reach up into Touchdown.

➤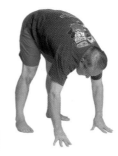

2
FORWARD BEND
Exhale as you fold forward.

➤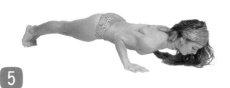

5
LOWER DOWN
Lower your body down slowly 3 . . . 2 . . . 1 while you squeeze your elbows in toward your ribs, making sure that your shoulders don't dip below your elbows. Now hover three inches off the mat, if possible, and hold 3 . . . 2 . . . 1. Then fully exhale and lower yourself to the mat.

➤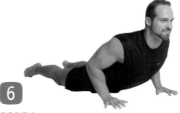

6
COBRA
Inhale and lengthen into Cobra by pressing your palms into the floor, lifting your chest, and rolling your shoulders back.

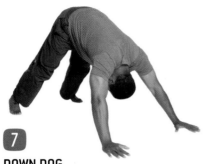

7

DOWN DOG

Exhale and push back into Down Dog by lifting your hips and pushing your chest back toward your feet while you take two small steps forward. Take one deep inhalation.

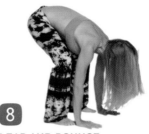

8

LEAP AND POUNCE

Exhale as you step or jump with both of your feet right behind your hands, keeping your knees bent.

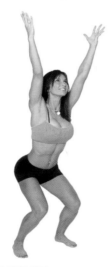

11

THUNDERBOLT

Inhale as you lift your ass, chest, shoulders, and arms skyward while you squeeze your knees a little closer. Now look up at your hands, and pretend you're sitting on a chair.

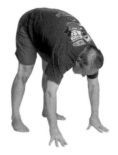

12

FORWARD BEND

Exhale, straighten your legs, and hang forward.

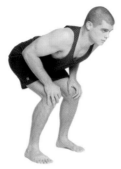

➤ 9

BARBACK

Inhale, slide your hands up to your knees, flatten your back, and press your heels out slightly.

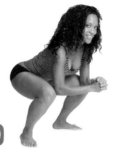

➤ 10

CATCHER'S POSITION

Exhale, drop, and squat. See if you can keep your heels flat on the floor, and pull your knees toward each other.

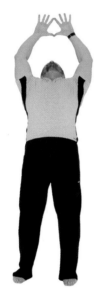

➤ 13

DIAMOND CUTTER

Inhale, and come on up with a flat back and arms wide. Tighten your belly and reach your arms to the sky, making the Diamond Cutter Sign while arching back.

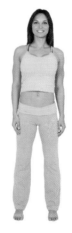

➤ 14

MOUNTAIN POSITION

Exhale and feel the BANG as you lower your hands to your sides.

Repeat this sequence two more times.

WINGS AND THINGS

This section keeps the heat going while working the quads, hip flexors, and upper body. "Wings and Things" is designed to reverse the adverse effects of too much wings and beer. The **Lunge Position** and **Modified Warrior** increase strength, flexibility, and balance in the presence of the burn. We also divided the Modified Warrior into different phases so that you can work on this position at the level you're most comfortable. It will give you something to work toward if you can't complete all phases initially. The **Lunge Twist** wrings out tension and toxins in the back, chest, and shoulders. Now go get ya some!

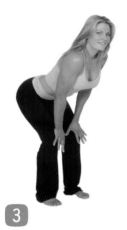

3

BARBACK
Inhale, bend your knees, slide your hands up to your knees, lift your head, and roll your shoulders back. Slide your heels out a bit, and feel your hips open.

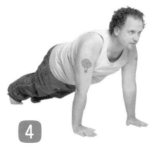

4

PUSH-UP POSITION
Lower your hands to the mat, and step or jump back into a push-up position.

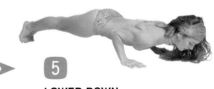

5

LOWER DOWN
Lower your body down slowly 3 . . . 2 . . . 1 while you squeeze your elbows in toward your ribs, making sure that your shoulders don't dip below your elbows. Now hover three inches off the mat and hold, if possible, for a count of 3 . . . 2 . . . 1. Then fully exhale and lower yourself to the mat.

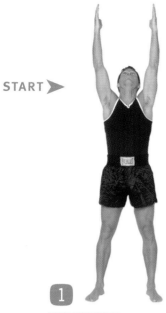

1 TOUCHDOWN
Inhale as you reach up into Touchdown.

➤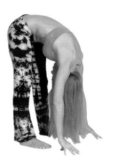

2 FORWARD BEND
Exhale and fold forward.

➤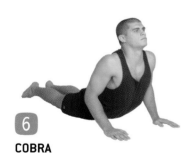

6 COBRA
Inhale and lengthen into Cobra by pressing your palms into the floor, lifting your chest, and rolling your shoulders back.

➤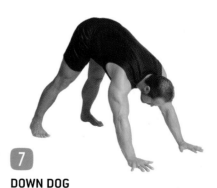

7 DOWN DOG
Exhale and push back into Down Dog by lifting your hips and pushing your chest back toward your feet while you take two small steps forward.

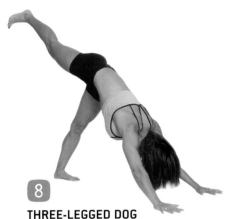

8
THREE-LEGGED DOG
Inhale and raise your right leg way up to the sky.

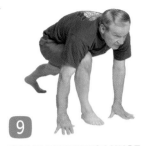

9
RIGHT RUNNER'S LUNGE
Exhale and swing that right leg forward, placing your right ankle directly below your knee.

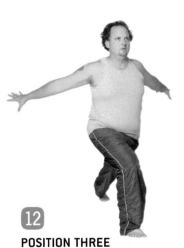

12
POSITION THREE
Inhale and swing your arms back like wings. Keep them back as if you are holding a big Theraball behind you.

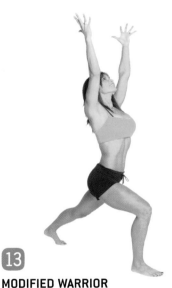

13
MODIFIED WARRIOR
On the next inhalation, if you can, reach your arms to the sky, squeeze your shoulders back, lift your chest, and look up at your hands. Take two more deep inhalations and exhalations.

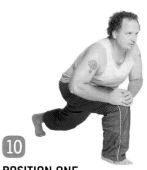

10

POSITION ONE
Inhale and place your hands on your right knee, with your left leg reaching straight back.

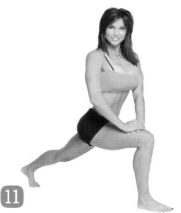

11

POSITION TWO
On your next inhalation, straighten your arms on that right knee while lifting your chest and squeezing your shoulders back.

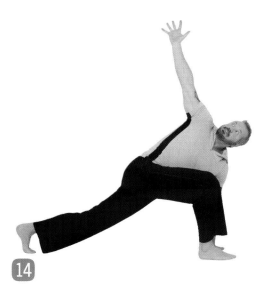

14

LUNGE TWIST
Exhale and lower your left hand to the floor while reaching your right hand to the sky. Pull your right knee closer to your chest. Reach higher on each inhalation. Open that right shoulder and twist more deeply on each exhalation. Take three deep breaths.

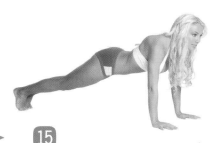

15

PUSH-UP POSITION
Exhale, drop your right hand to the floor, swing your right leg back, and move into a push-up position.

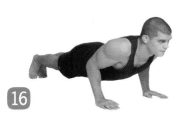

16 LOWER DOWN

Lower your body down slowly 3 . . . 2 . . . 1 as you squeeze your elbows in toward your ribs, making sure that your shoulders don't dip below your elbows. Now hover three inches off the mat and hold, if possible, for a count of 3 . . . 2 . . . 1. Then fully exhale and lower yourself to the mat.

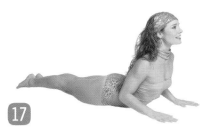

17 COBRA

Inhale and lengthen into Cobra by pressing your palms into the floor, lifting your chest, and rolling your shoulders back.

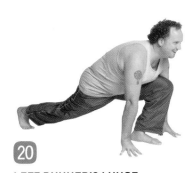

20 LEFT RUNNER'S LUNGE

Exhale and swing that left leg forward into a lunge position with your left ankle directly below your knee.

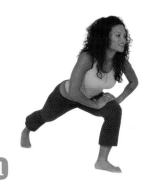

21 POSITION ONE

Inhale and place your hands on your left knee.

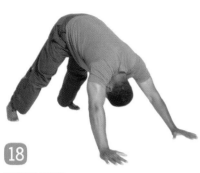

➤ **18**

DOWN DOG
Exhale and push back into Down Dog by lifting your hips and pushing your chest back toward your feet while you take two small steps forward.

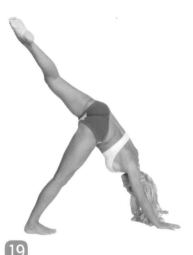

➤ **19**

THREE-LEGGED DOG
Inhale and raise your left leg way up high.

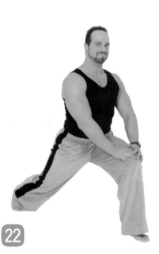

➤ **22**

POSITION TWO
On your next inhalation, lift your head and chest up into Position Two.

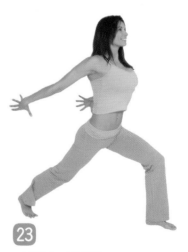

➤ **23**

POSITION THREE
Inhale again and take flight as you swing your arms back like wings.

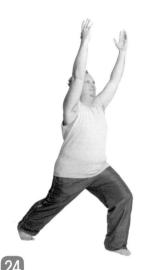

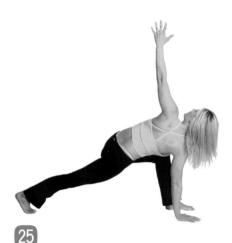

24

MODIFIED WARRIOR

On the next inhalation, reach your arms to the sky, squeeze your shoulders back, lift your chest, and look up at your hands, moving into Modified Warrior if you can. Take two more deep breaths.

25

LUNGE TWIST

Exhale and lower your right hand to the floor while reaching your left hand to the sky in a Lunge Twist. Pull your left knee closer to your chest. Reach higher on each inhalation. Open that left shoulder and twist more deeply on each exhalation. Take three deep breaths.

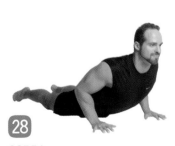

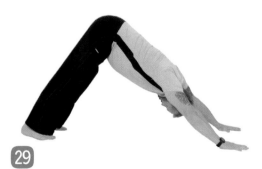

28

COBRA

Inhale and lengthen into Cobra.

29

DOWN DOG

Exhale and push back into Down Dog. Take a deep inhalation.

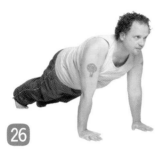

26

PUSH-UP POSITION

Exhale, drop your left hand to the floor, swing your left leg back, and move into a push-up position.

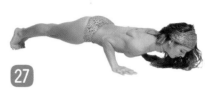

27

LOWER DOWN

Lower your body down slowly 3 . . . 2 . . . 1 while you squeeze your elbows in toward your ribs, making sure that your shoulders don't dip below your elbows. Now hover three inches off the mat, and hold, if possible, for a count of 3 . . . 2 . . . 1. Then, fully exhale and lower yourself to the mat.

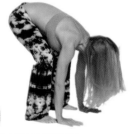

30

LEAP AND POUNCE

Exhale as you step or jump with both of your feet right behind your hands, keeping your knees bent.

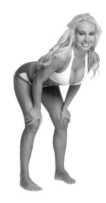

31

BARBACK

Inhale as you move up into Barback.

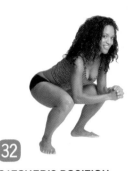

32

CATCHER'S POSITION

Exhale, drop, and squat into Catcher's Position.

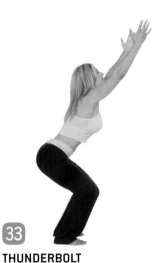

33

THUNDERBOLT

Inhale as you lift your ass, chest, shoulders, and arms skyward while you squeeze your knees a little closer. Now look up at your hands.

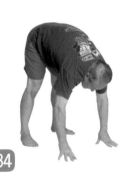

34

FORWARD BEND

Exhale, straighten your legs, and hang forward.

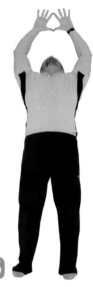

35

DIAMOND CUTTER

Inhale, and come on up with a flat back and arms wide. Tighten your belly and reach your arms to the sky. Make the Diamond Cutter Sign while arching back.

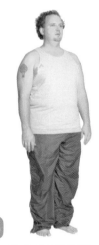

36

MOUNTAIN POSITION

Exhale and feel the BANG as you lower your hands to your sides.

MEET THE WARRIOR

We keep it all going with another modified Sun Salutation that introduces the traditional **Warrior One,** which places your back foot flat on the ground while you reach for the sky. This stretches and stabilizes your hips as you square those hips. We also continue our slow-motion burn with even more old school push-ups and controlled negative push-ups, which will increase your heart rate and your power.

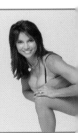

START ➤

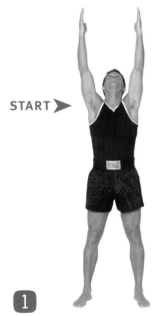

> **HOT TIP!**
> Are you ready to meet the position that can kick your ass? If you are having any trouble, it's okay. Take it slow, and if you need to, just use the modified positions from the last section by keeping your heel up.

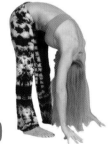

1
TOUCHDOWN
Inhale and reach up into Touchdown.

➤ **2**
FORWARD BEND
Exhale and fold forward.

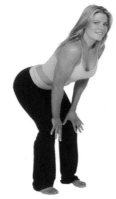

3

BARBACK

Inhale, bend your knees, slide your hands up to your knees, lift your head, and roll your shoulders back. Slide your heels out a bit and feel your hips open.

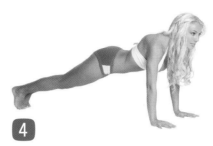

4

PUSH-UP POSITION

Lower your hands to the mat, and step or jump back into a push-up position.

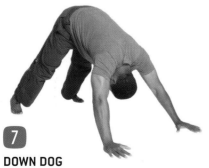

7

DOWN DOG

Exhale and push back into Down Dog by lifting your hips and pushing your chest back toward your feet while you take two small steps forward.

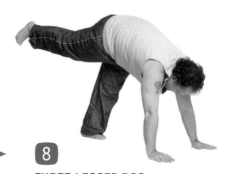

8

THREE-LEGGED DOG

Inhale, raise your right leg up high, push it way back, and feel the spinal traction.

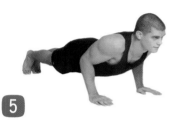

> **5**

LOWER DOWN

Lower your body down slowly 3 ... 2 ... 1 as you squeeze your elbows in toward your ribs, making sure that your shoulders don't dip below your elbows. Now hover three inches off the mat and hold, if possible, for a count of 3 ... 2 ... 1. Then fully exhale and lower yourself to the mat.

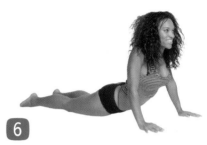

> **6**

COBRA

Inhale as you lengthen into Cobra by pressing your palms into the floor, lifting your chest, and rolling your shoulders back.

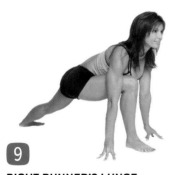

> **9**

RIGHT RUNNER'S LUNGE

Exhale, swing your right foot forward and place it so your right ankle is directly below your knee. Place your left foot flat.

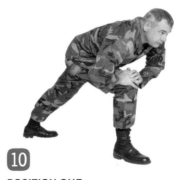

> **10**

POSITION ONE

Inhale and place both hands on your right knee.

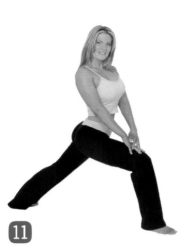

11

POSITION TWO

On your next inhalation, straighten your arms on that knee while lifting your chest and squeezing your shoulders.

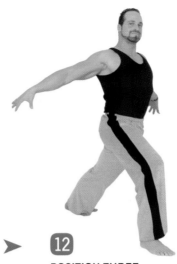

12

POSITION THREE

Inhale and take flight as you swing your arms back like wings. Keep them back as if you are holding a big Theraball behind you.

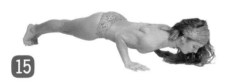

15

LOWER DOWN

Lower your body down slowly 3 . . . 2 . . . 1 as you squeeze your elbows in toward your ribs, making sure that your shoulders don't dip below your elbows. Now hover three inches off the mat, if possible, and hold for a count of 3 . . . 2 . . . 1. Then fully exhale and lower yourself to the mat.

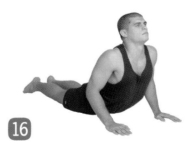

16

COBRA

Inhale and lengthen into Cobra.

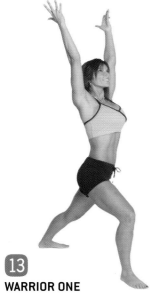

➤ ## 13 WARRIOR ONE
On your next inhalation, level your hips, bend your right knee deeper, and reach your arms to the sky while you squeeze your shoulders back, lift your chest, and look up at your hands. Take two more deep breaths.

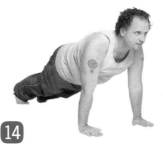

➤ ## 14 PUSH-UP POSITION
Exhale and move into a push-up position.

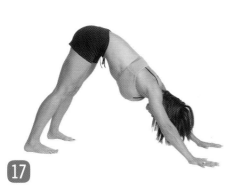

➤ ## 17 DOWN DOG
Exhale and push back into Down Dog.

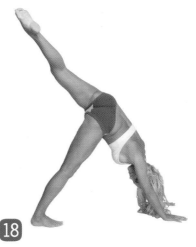

➤ ## 18 THREE-LEGGED DOG
Inhale and raise your left leg up high, push it way back, and feel the spinal traction.

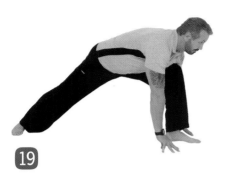

19

LEFT RUNNER'S LUNGE

Exhale, swing your left foot forward and place it so your left ankle is directly below your knee. Place your right foot flat.

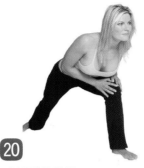

20

POSITION ONE

Inhale and place both hands on your left knee.

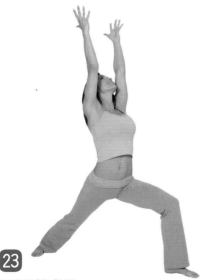

23

WARRIOR ONE

Inhale, level your hips, bend your left knee deeper, and reach your arms to the sky while you squeeze your shoulders back. Lift your chest and look up at your hands. Take two more deep breaths.

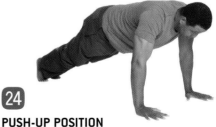

24

PUSH-UP POSITION

Exhale, lower your hands to the mat, and step or jump back into a push-up position.

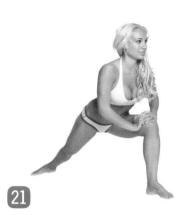

21

POSITION TWO

Inhale and straighten your arms on that left knee while lifting your chest and squeezing your shoulders back.

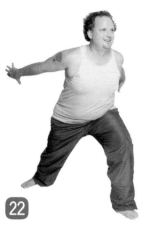

22

POSITION THREE

Inhale and take flight again as you swing your arms back.

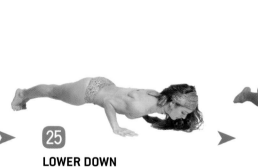

25

LOWER DOWN

Lower your body down slowly 3 . . . 2 . . . 1 while you squeeze your elbows in toward your ribs. Hover three inches off the mat, and hold for 3 . . . 2 . . . 1. Then fully exhale and lower yourself to the mat.

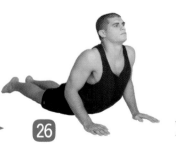

26

COBRA

Inhale and lengthen into Cobra.

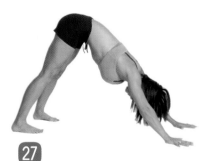

27

DOWN DOG

Exhale and push back into Down Dog.

BRING IT ON HOME

Now we've turned the corner and we're ready to begin our cool-down. We put more **Cat Lifts** and **Cat Arches** in this section because you can really work the kinks out of your spine when you're good and hot. It's also a great time for you to steal a "butt shot" glimpse of the yoga-babes nearby. The Cat Lift and the Cat Arch make for some beautiful scenery! Hell, if that won't keep you motivated to hang in there, you're dead! I guarantee this sequence will awaken your spine, get the blood flowing, and get you movin' right!

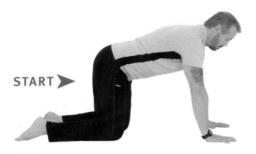

START ➤

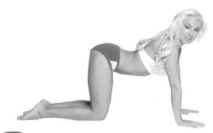

1 **TABLE TOP**
Exhale, drop your knees and your hands to the floor, and move to Table Top.

2 **CAT LIFT**
Inhale, lift your head, roll your shoulders back, and fill your belly with breath.

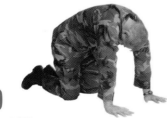

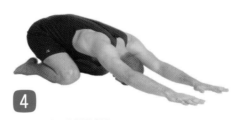

3 **CAT ARCH**
Exhale, drop your head, round your spine, and look back at your belly button. Repeat Cat Lift to Cat Arch two more times.

4 **CHILD'S POSITION**
Push back into Child's Position by reaching your arms forward and pushing your hips back toward your heels. Lower your forehead toward the floor and feel the spinal traction. Take three deep breaths.

GO HOME
The Closing Sequence

Check your racing forms, guys, because we're into the home stretch! The **Dead Bug** looks more like a **Happy Porn Star**, but no matter how you name it, it's a killer hip, back, and groin stretch. The **Bridge Position** puts you back together by resetting your back muscles after all that forward bending. It's also a great low back and pelvis training tool so you can satisfy your happy porn star. The **Easy Twist** wrings out that last bit of tension from your low back.

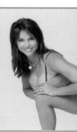

> **HOT TIP!**
> This is one great post-workout cool-down. It's also a great way to stretch out before you dismount from your bed. It incorporates flexions, extensions, hip stabilizers, hip openers, and twists for a perfectly balanced mini-workout.

START ➤

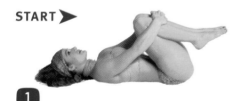

1
KNEES TO CHEST
Roll onto your back, pull your knees into your chest, and let your neck and shoulders relax to the floor. Take three deep breaths.

➤

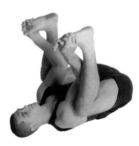

2
DEAD BUG
Release your legs, let the soles of your feet face the sky, grab the outside of each foot, and pull the knees toward the ground into Dead Bug. Take three deep breaths.

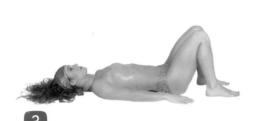

3
PINFALL
Drop your feet flat to the floor with knees bent.

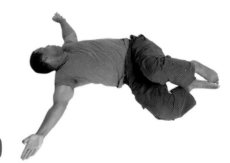

4
EASY TWIST
Let your knees drop to the right and look over your left shoulder. Inhale deeply and pull your knees even further to the right as you exhale into the twist. Take three deep breaths.

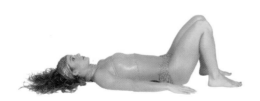

7
PINFALL
Drop your feet flat to the floor with knees bent.

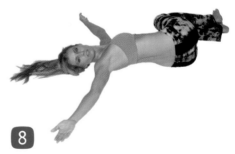

8
EASY TWIST
Let your knees drop to the left and look over your right shoulder. Inhale deeply and pull your knees even further to the left as you exhale. Take three deep breaths.

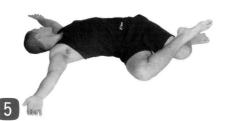

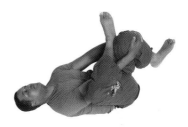

➤ **5**

DEEPER TWIST

Cross your right ankle over your left knee, keep your shoulders flat, and increase the stretch in your hips by guiding that left knee to the floor with your right ankle. Take three deep breaths.

➤ **6**

CROSS-LEGGED STRETCH

Inhale while the right ankle is still crossed over your left knee. Pull your left knee toward your chest, and grab the left knee with both hands, coming into the Cross-Legged Stretch. Relax your neck and shoulders as you try to let your tailbone touch the floor. Take three deep breaths.

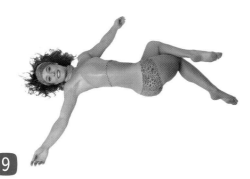

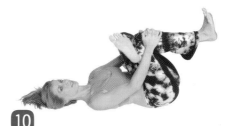

➤ **9**

DEEPER TWIST

Cross your left ankle over your right knee, keep your shoulders flat, and increase the stretch in your hips by guiding the right knee to the floor. Take three deep breaths.

➤ **10**

CROSS-LEGGED STRETCH

Inhale. While your left ankle is still crossed over your right knee, pull that right knee toward your chest and grab your right knee with both hands, coming back into Cross-Legged Stretch. Relax your neck and shoulders while you try to let your tailbone touch the floor. Take three deep breaths.

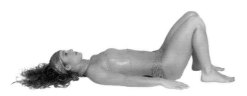

 11

PINFALL

Exhale and drop both feet flat on the floor.

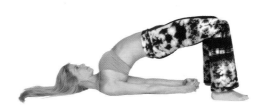

 12

BRIDGE POSITION

Inhale, and with bent knees, lift your hips up into Bridge Position. Squeeze your knees toward each other, and squeeze your shoulder blades together for stability as you clasp hands and press your fists down toward your feet. Lift your chest a little higher on each inhalation. Take three deep breaths.

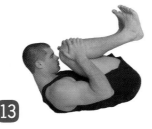

13

THE HUMAN BALL

Exhale and drop your hips to the floor; then squeeze your knees up into your chest as you pull your head up toward your knees. Stay for three deep breaths, as we counter a strong extension position with a deep flexion position.

THE FINISH
Ring the Bell, It's Over!

This is where you get the payoff. This position helps your body digest and assimilate all of the work you've just done over the last twenty minutes. "The Finish" turns this workout into something useful for your body and your mind.

If you do this 20-Minute Workout three days a week, it will change your life. Now if you want to take it to the next level, try the 30-Minute Workout on the next page and you'll really start to burn some fat off your jelly belly and those industrial-strength love handles.

START ➤ ZZZZZZZZZZZZZZZZZZZZZZ . . .

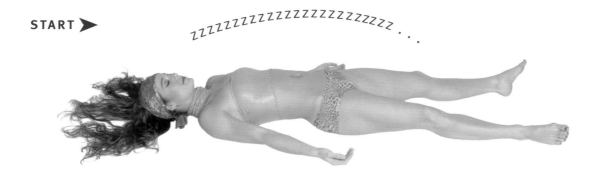

TOTALLY RELAX
Straighten your legs, pin your shoulders to your mat, and let your hands fall by your sides with the palms facing up. Now we will count how many deep, long, slow belly breaths we can take through our nose before we pass out and snore. Relax your neck and TOTALLY RELAX for five to ten minutes.

30 ›MINUTE WORKOUT SECTIONS

IGNITION

FIRE UP THE BACK AND HIPS

TOUCHDOWNS AND SIDE BENDS

RAINING CATS, DOGS, AND COBRAS

BROKEN TABLE PLUS NEW!

GET HOT

WINGS AND THINGS

MEET THE WARRIOR

SWEAT YOUR ASS OFF NEW!

BRING IT ON HOME

GO HOME

THE FINISH

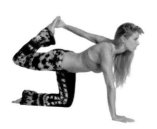
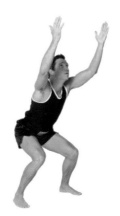
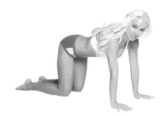

MINUTE WORKOUT

I know a lot of you hate the StairMaster, the treadmill, or the bike. You hate doggin' it down the block. What if I told you that by adding just ten minutes to what you are already doing, you can increase your cardiovascular strength and endurance, as well as your fat-burning capacity? I'm not bullshitting you—ten more minutes will do just that.

In this workout you're going to use your 20-Minute Workout foundation and add a few extra moves to turn up the heat and keep it interesting. Yoga-Doc and I added these particular positions because we wanted to guide you more deeply into the cardio world of YRG. The 20-Minute Workout is designed to get you warmed up and make some gains in flexibility. The 30-Minute Workout is *guaranteed* to make you sweat. In fact, the new sequence "Sweat Your Ass Off" delivers as advertised by introducing you to four new positions that are the foundation for most power yoga workouts.

The "Broken Table Plus" sequence adds a great new position that will challenge your hips and glutes; at the same time, it will keep your heart rate up. In each of these yoga positions, you need to remember to engage, flex, and tighten your muscles up onto your long bones to enhance your heart rate and create an isometric-strength workout at the same time.

Now look on the bright side: You don't have to do all those pain-in-the-ass cardio machines anymore. You can do this workout anywhere, and you only need enough room to do a push-up. The benefit of adding more time to your workout is *endurance*. The more time you can fit into your workout, the stronger, leaner, and younger you'll feel.

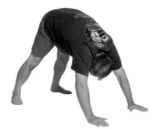

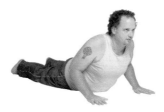

BROKEN TABLE PLUS

By substituting this sequence for the 20-Minute Workout's "Broken Table" (p. 42), we added a little extra heat with the **Awkward Airplane**. Enjoy!

(p. 42)

START ▸

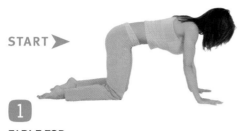

1
TABLE TOP
Inhale and move to Table Top.

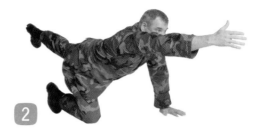

2
RIGHT TABLE TOP TRACTION
Now raise your left leg straight back with intention while reaching your right arm straight ahead, as if stretching out to shake someone's hand. Take three deep breaths while you engage your arm muscles and leg muscles strongly.

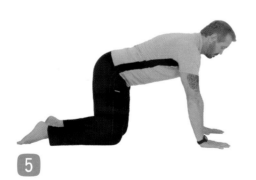

5
TABLE TOP
Exhale, and move back into Table Top.

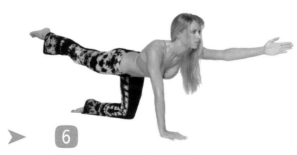

6
LEFT TABLE TOP TRACTION
Inhale and switch to the opposite side. Lift and push your right leg straight back while you strongly reach your left arm straight ahead. Take three deep breaths.

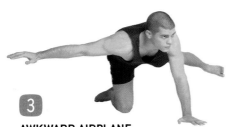

➤ **3**

AWKWARD AIRPLANE

Now bring your left leg out to the left, and straighten it if you can. Bring that right arm out to the right. Take three deep breaths as you pull your belly in and concentrate on your balance. Feel your ass catch fire!

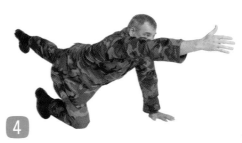

➤ **4**

RIGHT TABLE TOP TRACTION

Reach forward again with your right arm and push that left leg straight back behind you. Take three deep breaths.

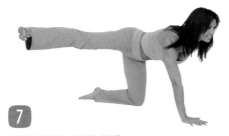

➤ **7**

AWKWARD AIRPLANE

Now bring your right leg out to the right and straighten it if you can. Bring that left arm out to the left. Take three deep breaths. While you press that right hand into the floor, engage your core and feel the Bunsen Burner.

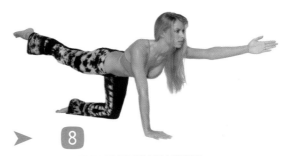

➤ **8**

LEFT TABLE TOP TRACTION

Reach forward again with your left arm and push that right leg back behind you. Take three deep breaths.

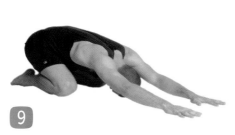

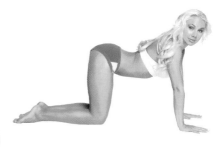

9

CHILD'S POSITION

Exhale and push your ass back toward your heels while reaching your arms far forward; rest your forehead on the ground. Take three deep breaths.

10

CAT LIFT

Inhale and return to Cat Lift.

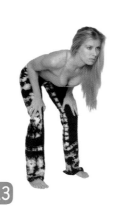

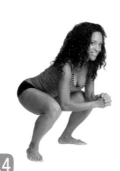

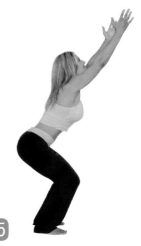

13

BARBACK

Inhale, slide your hands up to your knees, flatten your back, and press your heels out slightly.

14

CATCHER'S POSITION

Exhale and squat into Catcher's Position. See if you can keep your heels flat on the floor.

15

THUNDERBOLT

Inhale and lift your chest, shoulders, and arms skyward while squeezing your knees a little closer. Now look up at your hands.

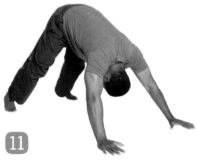

11

DOWN DOG

Exhale, push your hips up, and straighten your arms as you press back into Down Dog. Take one deep inhalation.

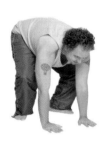

12

LEAP AND POUNCE

Exhale and step or jump right behind your hands with bent knees.

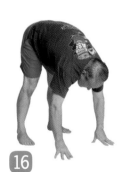

16

FORWARD BEND

Exhale, straighten your legs, and hang forward.

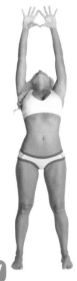

17

DIAMOND CUTTER

Inhale and come up with a flat back and arms wide. Tighten your belly and reach your arms to the sky, making the Diamond Cutter Sign and arching back.

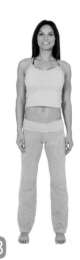

18

MOUNTAIN POSITION

Exhale and feel the BANG as you lower your hands to your sides.

SWEAT YOUR ASS OFF

This section is the meat and potatoes of the 30-Minute Workout. It's where we wear you out with some seriously strong standing positions that will challenge your strength, stamina, flexibility, and pain tolerance. **Warrior Two** is a good pose for leg strength and good posture. **Reverse Warrior** opens your rib cage, shoulders, and lung fields while your lower body is strengthened and stretched. **Extended Side Angle** is another all-in-one position that stretches and strengthens your legs, glutes, back, sides, shoulders, and neck. It opens you up from the inside out! And the **Triangle** tests your balance while stretching your hamstrings, back, and shoulders.

HOT TIP!
You had better "hulk up," guys, because this one is a slobber-knocker! Oh, one more thing—keep your breathing steady and your focus like a samurai, because this is the hard part!

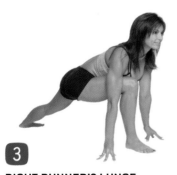

▼ 3

RIGHT RUNNER'S LUNGE
Exhale and swing your right foot forward. Your right ankle should be placed directly below that right knee. Keep your left foot flat on the floor.

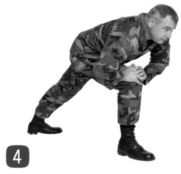

➤ 4

POSITION ONE
Inhale and place both hands on your right knee.

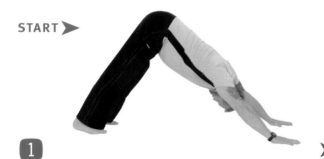

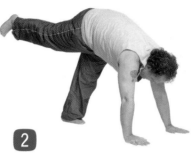

1
DOWN DOG
Exhale and push back into Down Dog by lifting your hips and pushing your chest back toward your feet.

2
THREE-LEGGED DOG
Inhale, raise your right leg up high, and push it way back.

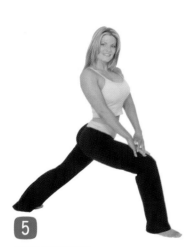

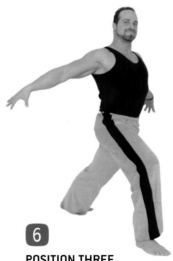

5
POSITION TWO
On your next inhalation, straighten your arms on that knee, lift your chest, and squeeze your shoulders back.

6
POSITION THREE
Inhale, swing your arms back like wings, and keep them back as if you are holding a big Theraball behind you.

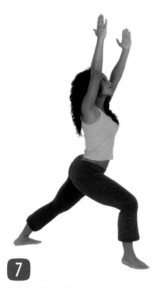

7

➤

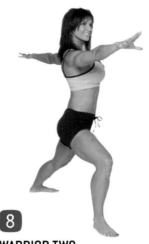

8

WARRIOR ONE

On the next inhalation, reach your arms to the sky, squeeze your shoulders back, lift your chest, and look up at your hands. Take two deep breaths.

WARRIOR TWO

Exhale as you bring your right arm forward and your left arm back. Strongly engage your arm and leg muscles to your bones as you look over the fingertips of your right hand and come into Warrior Two. Take three deep breaths.

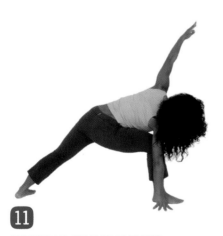

▼

11

➤

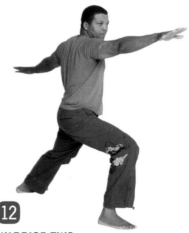

12

EXTENDED SIDE ANGLE TWO

Exhale, roll your left shoulder back more deeply, and try to place your right hand on the floor just to the right of your ankle. Take two more deep breaths.

WARRIOR TWO

Inhale and pull back up into Warrior Two. Take three deep breaths.

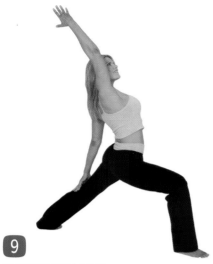

9

REVERSE WARRIOR

Inhale, slide your left hand down your left leg, and raise your right hand to the sky while you bend your right knee deeply. Take three deep breaths.

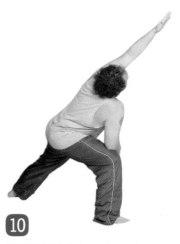

10

EXTENDED SIDE ANGLE ONE

Exhale, drop your right elbow onto your bent right knee, roll your left shoulder back, and raise your left arm above your ear. Inhale and look up at your left hand as you squeeze your belly in.

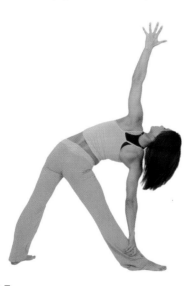

13

TRIANGLE

Exhale, straighten your right leg, reach your right arm forward, and place your right hand down your right knee or shin. Inhale, raise your left arm to the sky, and exhale as you roll that left shoulder back, keeping your head in direct alignment with your right foot. Take two more deep breaths.

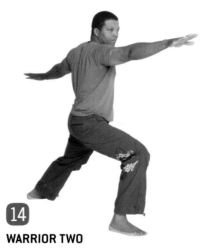

14

WARRIOR TWO

Inhale, and lift back up into Warrior Two. Take three deep breaths.

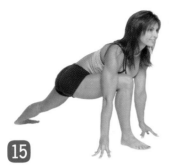

15

CARTWHEEL INTO LUNGE
Swing your right arm forward, followed by your left arm, and come into a lunge.

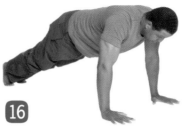

16

PUSH-UP POSITION
Exhale, and step back into a push-up position.

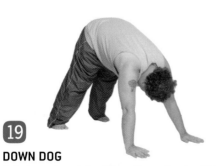

19

DOWN DOG
Exhale and push back into Down Dog by lifting your hips and pushing your chest back toward your feet while you take two small steps forward.

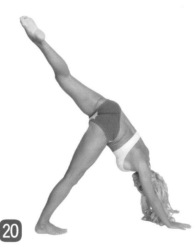

20

THREE-LEGGED DOG
Inhale, raise your left leg up high, and push it way back.

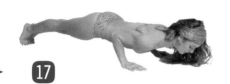

17
LOWER DOWN

Lower your body down slowly 3 . . . 2 . . . 1 as you squeeze your elbows in toward your ribs, making sure that your shoulders don't dip below your elbows. Now hover three inches off the mat and hold, if possible, for a count of 3 . . . 2 . . . 1. Then, fully exhale and lower yourself to the mat.

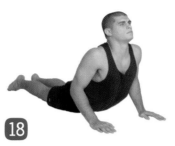

18
COBRA

Inhale and lengthen into Cobra. Press your palms into the floor, lift your chest, roll your shoulders back, and look up to the sky.

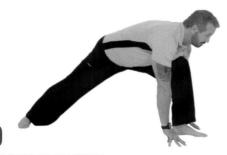

21
LEFT RUNNER'S LUNGE

Exhale, and swing your left foot forward, placing left ankle directly below the left knee and your right foot flat.

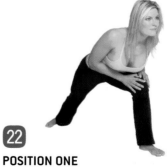

22
POSITION ONE

Inhale and place both hands on your left knee.

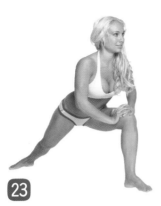

23

POSITION TWO
On your next inhalation, straighten your arms on that knee while lifting your chest and squeezing your shoulders back.

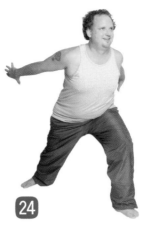

24

POSITION THREE
Inhale, swing your arms back like wings, and keep them back as if you are holding a big Theraball behind you.

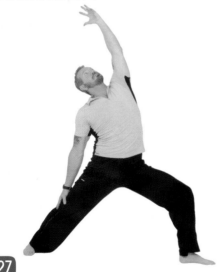

27

REVERSE WARRIOR
Inhale, slide your right hand down on your right knee, and raise your left hand to the sky while you bend your left knee deeply. Take three deep breaths.

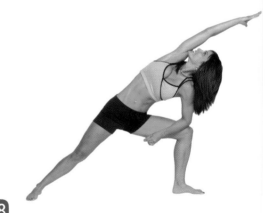

28

EXTENDED SIDE ANGLE ONE
Exhale, drop your left elbow onto your left knee, roll your right shoulder back, and raise your right arm over your ear. Inhale and look up at your right hand as you squeeze your belly in.

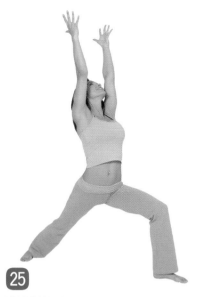

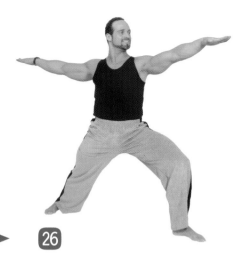

> **25**

WARRIOR ONE

On the next inhalation, reach your arms to the sky, squeeze your shoulders back, lift your chest, and look up at your hands. Take two deep breaths.

> **26**

WARRIOR TWO

Exhale as you bring your left arm forward and your right arm back. Strongly engage your arm and leg muscles to your bones as you look over the fingertips of your right hand and come into Warrior Two. Take three deep breaths.

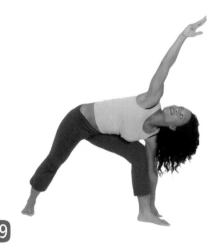

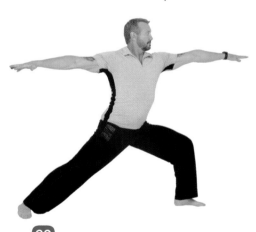

> **29**

EXTENDED SIDE ANGLE TWO

Exhale, roll your right shoulder back more deeply, and try to place your left hand on the floor, just to the left of your ankle. Take two more deep breaths.

> **30**

WARRIOR TWO

Inhale and pull back up into Warrior Two. Take three deep breaths.

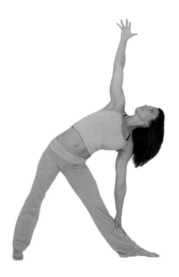

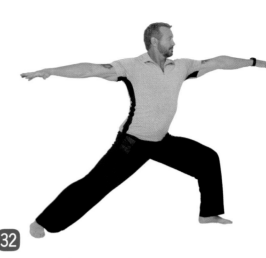

31
TRIANGLE

Exhale, straighten your left leg, reach your left arm forward, and place your left hand down your left knee or shin. Inhale, raise your right arm to the sky, and exhale as you roll that right shoulder back, keeping your head in direct alignment with your left foot. Take two more deep breaths.

32
WARRIOR TWO

Inhale as you bend your left knee and lift back up into Warrior Two. Take three deep breaths.

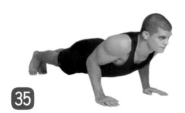

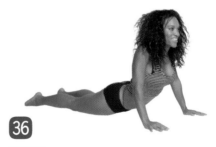

35
LOWER DOWN

Lower your body down slowly 3 . . . 2 . . . 1 as you squeeze your elbows in toward your ribs, making sure that your shoulders don't dip below your elbows. Now hover three inches off the mat and hold, if possible, for a count of 3 . . . 2 . . . 1. Then fully exhale and lower yourself to the mat.

36
COBRA

Inhale and lengthen into Cobra.

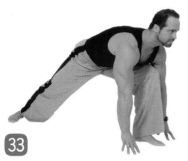

33

CARTWHEEL INTO LUNGE

Swing your left arm forward, followed by your right arm, and come into a lunge.

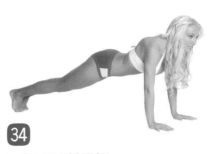

34

PUSH-UP POSITION

Lower your hands to the mat, and step or jump back into a push-up position.

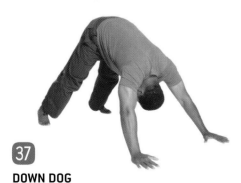

37

DOWN DOG

Exhale and push back into Down Dog. Take one deep inhalation.

Aerial Down Dog . . .

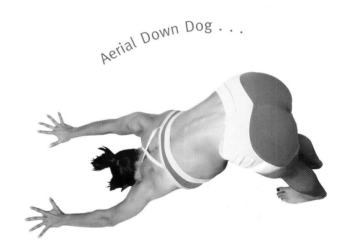

45 ›MINUTE WORKOUT SECTIONS

- IGNITION
- FIRE UP THE BACK AND HIPS
- TOUCHDOWNS AND SIDE BENDS
- RAINING CATS, DOGS, AND COBRAS
- FIX THE BROKEN TABLE NEW!
- GET HOT
- WINGS AND THINGS
- MEET THE WARRIOR
- SWEAT YOUR ASS OFF AND TWIST NEW!
- RUSSIAN LEG SWEEPS NEW!
- WRAP AND BURN NEW!
- OPEN YOUR CAN AND WALK THE PLANK NEW!
- BRING IT ON HOME
- GO HOME
- THE FINISH

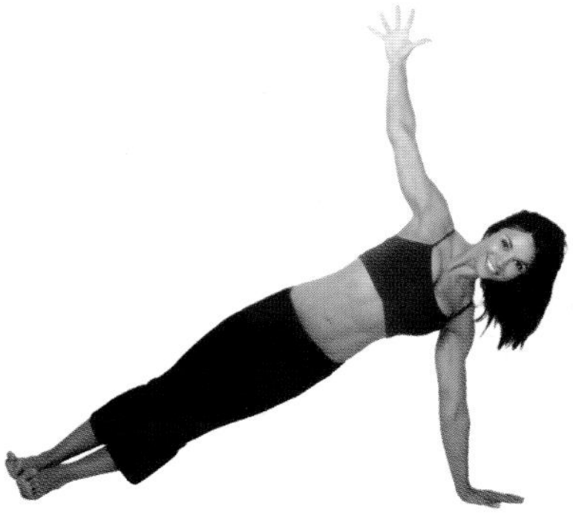

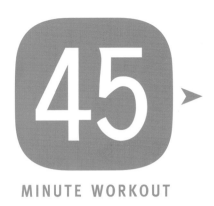

MINUTE WORKOUT

If you're up to this section, I want to tell you how proud of you I am! You're kicking ass, bro; as soon as you have completed this workout, I want you to go right to **www.diamonddallaspage.com** and sign up for the "Forty-Five and Over Club." You, my brother, are one of the **BIG DOGS**. This workout is geared to kick the Regular Guy's ass; you may even fall on your ass a time or two. (I know I did!) You know what? That's okay. Remember, it's not how many times you fall down that counts—it's how many times you get back up. We're still using the core regimens you've learned in the 20-Minute Workout and 30-Minute Workout. But now we've added some great new positions to challenge you and keep you entertained for another fifteen minutes.

We added an extra step to "Fix the Broken Table" that will test your balance and ability to focus. The position added to create "Sweat Your Ass Off and Twist" is a great one to challenge your balance along with your hip, shoulder, and chest flexibility. The "Russian Leg Sweeps" section is for knee strengthening and stability. "Wrap and Burn" is your initiation into the fraternity of pretzel-like positions, but you get to control how far you go. (This isn't a yoga hazing after all!) And "Open Your Can and Walk the Plank" is a combination of mack-daddy hip openers and a total body-strengthening position that might make you want to "tap out" (a wrestling term) the first time you try it.

In this workout we're going to push your strength, power, flexibility, and focus to a new level. Once you get this program down, you can move to the next chapter and add the heart accelerator section to really increase your heart rate. By doing so, you are not going to *believe* how much fat you are going to burn. This is where "sweat your ass off" takes on a whole new meaning. By adding time to your workout, you can choose the one that's right for you based on the time available, your level of experience, and your energy level on that particular day. Once you learn your base, your workout never has to be the same again. Now, if you're really ready to start—to quote my favorite Copenhagen-dippin', coupon-clippin', draft beer–drinkin' redneck, Stone Cold Steve Austin: "Give me a HELL YEAH!"

FIX THE BROKEN TABLE

In this section, we added an intermediate step to the Awkward Airplane that is both a quad stretch and a balance challenge. Don't pull on your knee too hard here— stay safe and relax.

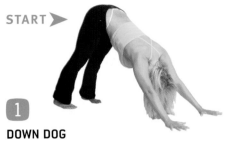

START ➤

1 DOWN DOG
Exhale and push back into Down Dog.

➤

2 TABLE TOP
Inhale and move back to Table Top.

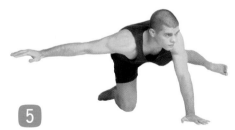

5 AWKWARD AIRPLANE
Now, straighten that left leg and swing it to the left while your right arm straightens to the right. Take three deep breaths while you pull your belly in and concentrate on balance. Feel your ass catch fire!

➤

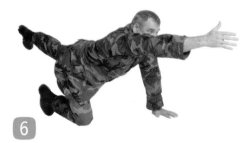

6 RIGHT TABLE TOP TRACTION
Reach forward again with your right arm and push that left leg straight back behind you. Take three deep breaths.

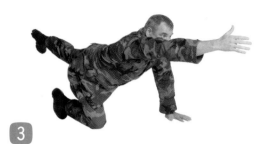

➤ **3**

RIGHT TABLE TOP TRACTION
Raise your left leg straight back with intention while reaching your right arm straight ahead as if stretching out to shake someone's hand. Take three deep breaths while you engage your arm muscles and leg muscles strongly.

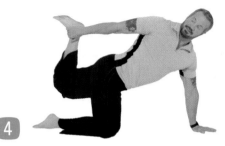

4

RIGHT TABLE TOP HOLD
Now, bend your left knee and grab your left ankle with your right hand. Take three deep breaths.

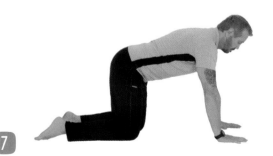

7

TABLE TOP
Exhale and move back into Table Top.

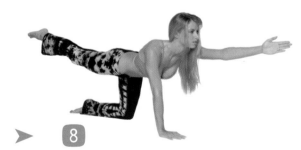

8

LEFT TABLE TOP TRACTION
Inhale, and move to the opposite side. Lift and push your right leg straight back while you strongly reach your left arm straight ahead. Take three deep breaths.

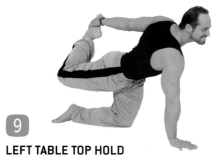

9

LEFT TABLE TOP HOLD
Now, slowly bend your right knee and grab your right ankle with your left hand. Take three deep breaths.

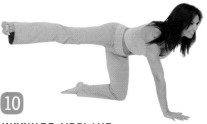

10

AWKWARD AIRPLANE
Now swing that right leg out to the right and straighten it while you bring your left arm out to the left. Take three deep breaths while you press that right hand into the floor, engage your core, and burn your butt.

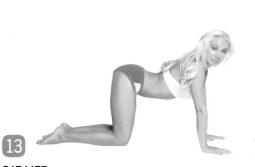

13

CAT LIFT
Inhale and return to Cat Lift.

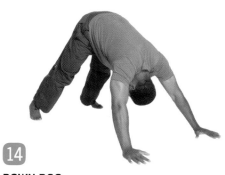

14

DOWN DOG
Exhale, curl your toes, push your hips up, and straighten your arms as you press back into Down Dog. Take a deep inhalation.

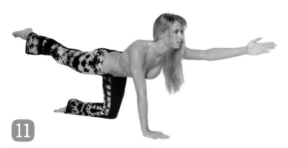

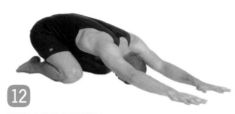

> **11**

LEFT TABLE TOP TRACTION
Reach forward again with your left arm and push that right leg back behind you. Take three deep breaths and hold your position.

> **12**

CHILD'S POSITION
Exhale, push your ass back toward your heels while reaching your arms far forward, and rest your head on the ground. Take three deep breaths.

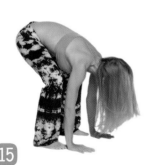

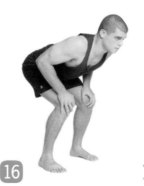

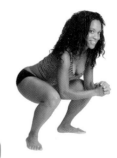

> **15**

LEAP AND POUNCE
Exhale and step or jump your feet right behind your hands, keeping your knees bent.

> **16**

BARBACK
Inhale, slide your hands up to your knees, flatten your back, and press your heels out slightly.

> **17**

CATCHER'S POSITION
Exhale as you drop and squat into Catcher's Position. See if you can keep your heels flat on the floor.

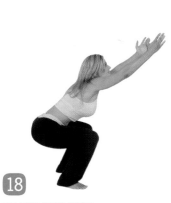

18

REACH AND RISE

Inhale as you lift your chest, shoulders, and arms skyward while you squeeze your knees a little closer.

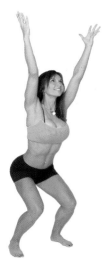

19

THUNDERBOLT

Now come into Thunderbolt and look up at your hands.

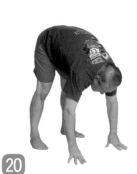

20

FORWARD BEND

Exhale, straighten your legs, and hang forward.

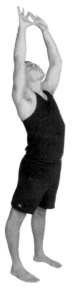

21

DIAMOND CUTTER

Inhale, come on up with a flat back and arms wide, tighten your belly, reach your arms to the sky, and make the Diamond Cutter Sign while arching back.

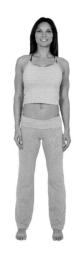

22

MOUNTAIN POSITION

Exhale and feel the BANG as you lower your arms back down to your sides.

SWEAT YOUR ASS OFF AND TWIST

This is the same killer section as the one in the 30-Minute Workout, except we added the **Twisted Triangle** for a little extra fun. Twisted Triangle works your hips, hamstrings, chest, shoulders, and neck. The twist massages the digestive system and internal organs, so it acts as a detoxifier. It also gives you a hell of a balance challenge. Go get it!

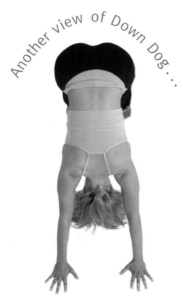

Another view of Down Dog...

START ➤

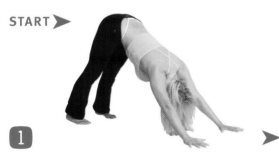

1
DOWN DOG
Exhale, curl your toes, push your hips up, and straighten your arms as you press back into Down Dog. Take a deep inhalation.

➤

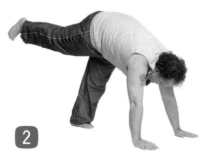

2
THREE-LEGGED DOG
Inhale, raise your right leg up high, and push it way back.

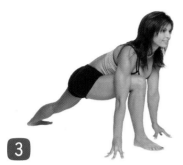

3

RIGHT RUNNER'S LUNGE

Exhale as you bring your right foot lunging forward, with your right ankle placed directly below that right knee. Place your left foot flat on the floor.

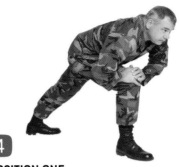

4

POSITION ONE

Inhale and place your hands on your right knee.

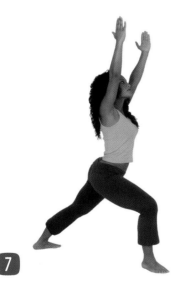

7

WARRIOR ONE

On the next inhalation, reach your arms to the sky, squeeze your shoulders back, lift your chest, and look up at your hands, coming into Warrior One. Take two deep breaths.

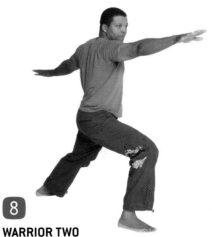

8

WARRIOR TWO

Exhale as you bring your right arm forward and your left arm back. Strongly engage your arm and leg muscles to your bones as you look over the fingertips of your right hand. Take three deep breaths.

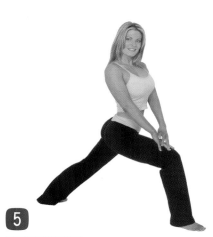

5

POSITION TWO

On your next inhalation, straighten your arms on that knee while lifting your chest and squeezing your shoulders back.

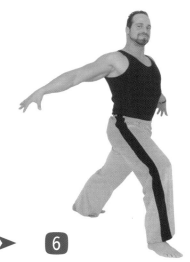

6

POSITION THREE

Inhale, swing your arms back like wings, and keep them back as if you are holding a big Theraball behind you.

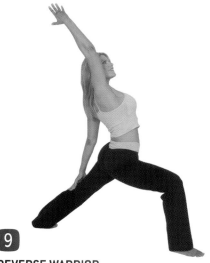

9

REVERSE WARRIOR

Inhale, slide your left hand down your left leg, and raise your right hand to the sky. Take three deep breaths.

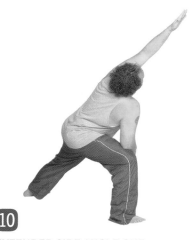

10

EXTENDED SIDE ANGLE ONE

Exhale, drop your right elbow onto your bent right knee, roll your left shoulder back, and raise your left arm above your ear. Take three deep breaths. Inhale and look up at your left hand as you squeeze your belly in.

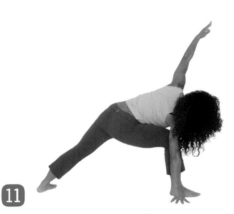

11

EXTENDED SIDE ANGLE TWO

Exhale, roll your left shoulder back more deeply, and see if you can place your right hand on the floor just to the right of your ankle as you take two more deep breaths.

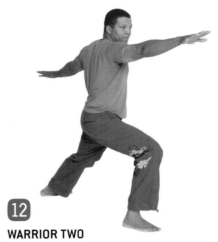

12

WARRIOR TWO

Inhale, pull back up into Warrior Two, and take three deep breaths.

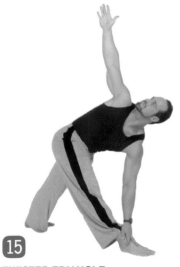

15

TWISTED TRIANGLE

Exhale, reach your left arm forward, and slide it down your right shin. Inhale, reach that right arm to the sky, push that right hip back, and press down into your left hand. Take three deep breaths.

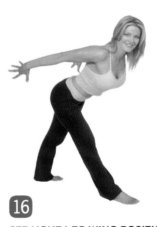

16

STRAIGHT LEG WING POSITION

Inhale and pull your torso up as you square your hips to the front. Swing your arms back in Wing Position.

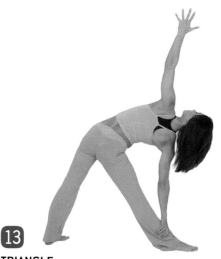

➤ **13**

TRIANGLE

Exhale, straighten your right leg, reach your right arm forward, and place your right hand down your right leg. Inhale, raise your left arm to the sky, and exhale. Roll that left shoulder back as you keep your head in direct alignment with your right foot. Take two more deep breaths.

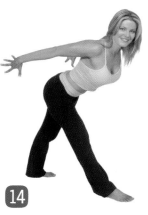

➤ **14**

STRAIGHT LEG WING POSITION

Now inhale and pull your torso up as you square your hips to the front. Swing your arms back in Wing Position.

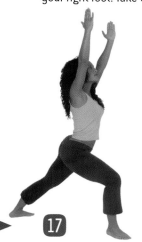

➤ **17**

WARRIOR ONE

On the next inhalation, bend your right knee, reach your arms to the sky, squeeze your shoulders back, lift your chest, and look up at your hands. Take two deep breaths.

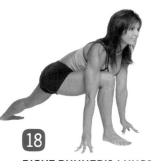

➤ **18**

RIGHT RUNNER'S LUNGE

Drop your hands to the floor and move to Right Runner's Lunge.

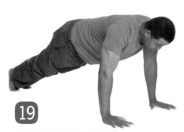

➤ **19**

PUSH-UP POSITION

Exhale, lower both hands to the mat, and step or jump back. Come into a push-up position.

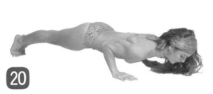

20

LOWER DOWN

Squeeze your elbows toward your ribs and don't let your chest drop below those elbows as you lower down 3 . . . 2 . . . 1, and hold 3 . . . 2 . . . 1.

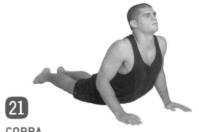

21

COBRA

Inhale and lengthen into Cobra.

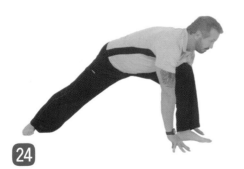

24

LEFT RUNNER'S LUNGE

Exhale as your left foot comes lunging forward, with your left ankle placed directly below that left knee. Keep your right foot flat on the floor.

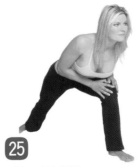

25

POSITION ONE

Inhale and place both hands on your left knee.

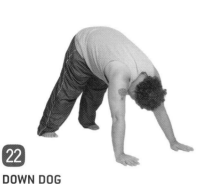

22

DOWN DOG
Exhale and push back into Down Dog.

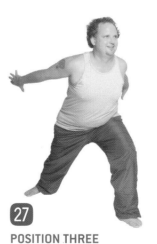

23

THREE-LEGGED DOG
Inhale, raise your left leg up high, and push it way back.

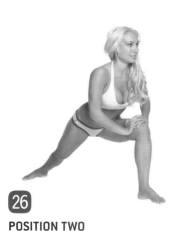

26

POSITION TWO
On your next inhalation, straighten your arms on that knee and lift your chest.

27

POSITION THREE
Inhale, swing your arms back like wings, and keep them back as if you are holding a big Theraball behind you.

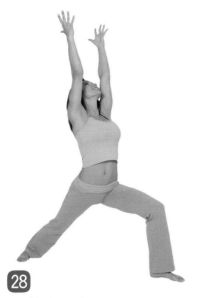

28

WARRIOR ONE

On the next inhalation, reach your arms to the sky, squeeze your shoulders back, lift your chest, and look up at your hands. Take two deep breaths.

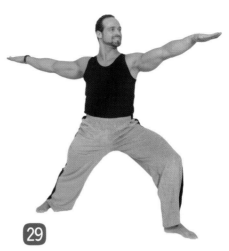

29

WARRIOR TWO

Exhale as you bring your left arm forward and your right arm back. Strongly engage your arm and leg muscles to your bones as you look over the fingertips of your right hand, and come into Warrior Two. Take three deep breaths.

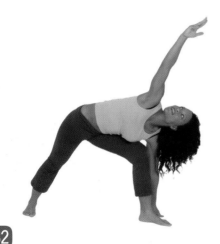

32

EXTENDED SIDE ANGLE TWO

Exhale, roll your right shoulder back more deeply, and see if you can place your left hand on the floor, just to the left of your ankle, coming into Extended Side Angle as you take two more deep breaths.

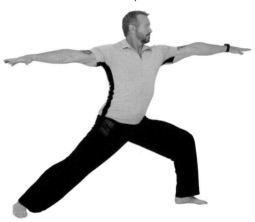

33

WARRIOR TWO

Inhale and pull back up into Warrior Two. Take three deep breaths.

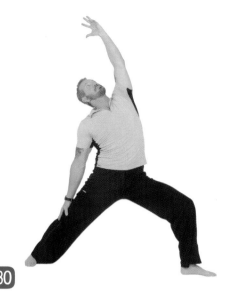

➤ **30**

REVERSE WARRIOR

Inhale, slide your right hand down your right leg, and raise your left hand to the sky while you bend your left knee deeply in Reverse Warrior. Take three deep breaths.

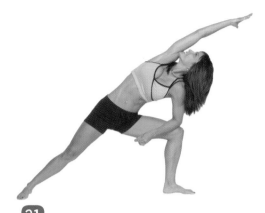

➤ **31**

EXTENDED SIDE ANGLE ONE

Exhale, drop your left elbow onto your bent left knee, roll your right shoulder back, and raise your right arm over your ear. Inhale and look up at your right hand as you squeeze your belly in.

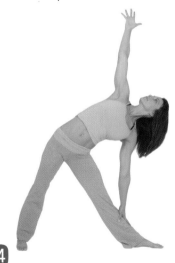

➤ **34**

TRIANGLE

Exhale, straighten your left leg, reach your left arm forward, and place your left hand down your left leg. Inhale, raise your right arm to the sky, and exhale. Roll that right shoulder back as you keep your head in direct alignment with your left foot. Take two more deep breaths.

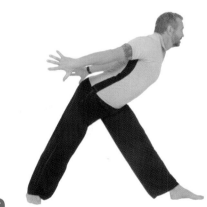

➤ **35**

STRAIGHT LEG WING POSITION

Now inhale and pull your torso up as you square your hips to the front. Swing your arms back in Wing Position.

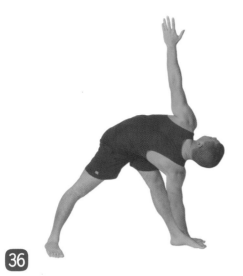

36

TWISTED TRIANGLE

Exhale, reach your right arm forward, and slide it down your left shin. Inhale, reach your left arm to the sky, push that left hip back, and press down into your right hand. Take three deep breaths.

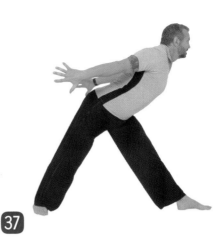

37

STRAIGHT LEG WING POSITION

Now inhale and pull your torso up as you square your hips to the front. Swing your arms back in Wing Position.

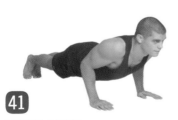

41

LOWER DOWN

Lower your body down slowly 3 . . . 2 . . . 1 while you squeeze your elbows in toward your ribs, making sure that your shoulders don't dip below your elbows. Now hover three inches off the mat, if possible, and hold 3 . . . 2 . . . 1. Then, fully exhale, and lower yourself to the mat.

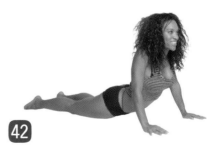

42

COBRA

Inhale and lengthen into Cobra.

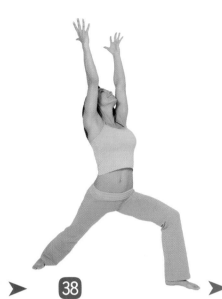

➤ **38**

WARRIOR ONE
On the next inhalation, bend your knee, reach your arms to the sky, squeeze your shoulders back, lift the chest, and look up at your hands. Take two deep breaths.

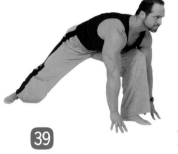

➤ **39**

LEFT RUNNER'S LUNGE
Drop your hands to the floor and move to Left Runner's Lunge.

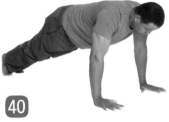

➤ **40**

PUSH-UP POSITION
Lower your hands to the mat, and step or jump back into a push-up position.

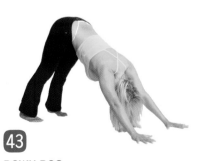

➤ **43**

DOWN DOG
Exhale and push back into Down Dog.

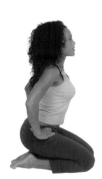

➤ **44**

RECOIL
Drop to your knees, place your hands on your hips, and slowly sit as far back toward your heels as you can.

RUSSIAN LEG SWEEPS

This section is a great knee strengthener. It is an adaptation on an old wrestling exercise called "knee walks" or "duck walks." It's all about moving your lower body to strengthen, stretch, and power up your quads while you build coordination and balance. And believe it or not, this will actually raise your heart rate to approximately 130 beats per minute or more—if done properly. Cheat 'til you don't have to cheat anymore! Whatever it takes, do it; you're building strength the entire time, and eventually, if you stay dedicated, you *won't* have to cheat anymore.

START ➤

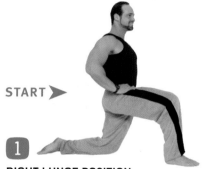

1
RIGHT LUNGE POSITION
Propelling yourself quickly from Recoil with hands on hips, inhale, sweep your right leg forward into a lunge position, and slowly count 3 . . . 2 . . . 1.

➤

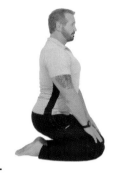

2
RECOIL
Exhale, sweep your right leg back, and sit back on your ankles as you lift your chest.

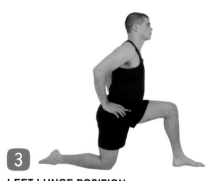

3
LEFT LUNGE POSITION
Inhale, sweep your left leg forward into a lunge position, and slowly count 3 . . . 2 . . . 1.

➤

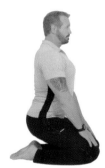

4
RECOIL
Exhale, sit back on your ankles, and lift your chest.

Repeat four more times, and drop back to your heels.

WRAP AND BURN

Get ready to experience a whole new level of YRG. Here we modify the **Extended Side Angle** position from a deep lunge and introduce a little bondage for some extra flavor. No, guys, I'm not talkin' whips and chains with yoga-babes in crotchless rubber suits—hmmm, maybe I should. I'm talking about the **Bound Extended Side Angle** position, which is the closest thing to a "pretzel position" that we'll have you do. It's a pure power pose that may remind you of the old school wrestling move called the "Abdominal Stretch." But in this case, you're inflicting it upon yourself.

Gird your loins and give it your best!

And here's a helpful hint: The more you relax and breathe while attempting to do this sequence, the more likely you'll be able to nail it. But remember, if you can't do it all, just do what you can, and you can try it again tomorrow. You may find it helpful to use a towel to lengthen your reach when you try to wrap your hands around your back. In time you will be able to clasp both hands behind your back.

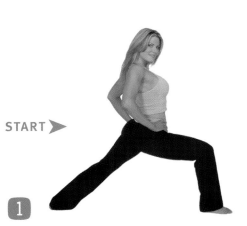

START ▶

1 **RIGHT LUNGE HANDS ON HIPS**
Using your momentum to propel yourself from Recoil, put your hands on your hips, inhale, and sweep your right foot forward into a lunge position and place your left foot flat.

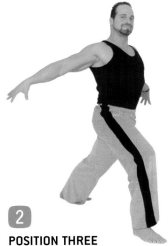

2 **POSITION THREE**
On your next inhalation, swing your arms back behind you and take flight.

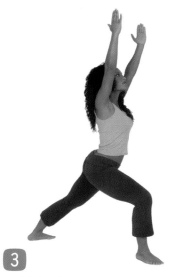

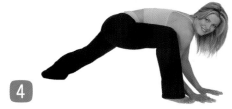

3
WARRIOR ONE

Inhale and reach your arms to the sky, squeeze your shoulders back, lift your chest, and look up at your hands in Warrior One.

4
LOW LUNGE

Exhale, drop down, and bring your hands to the inside of your right foot.

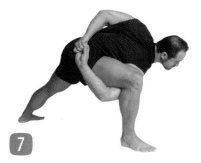

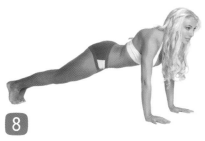

7
BOUND SIDE ANGLE THREE

Exhale, drop your left hand behind your back, and clasp those hands together in Bound Side Angle. Now inhale, squeeze your shoulder blades toward each other, keep those hands clasped behind you, and lean your head back. Try to take four more deep breaths.

8
PUSH-UP POSITION

Lower your hands to the mat, and step or jump back into a push-up position.

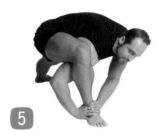

5

BOUND SIDE ANGLE ONE

Move your right arm beneath your right knee and see if you can grab your right ankle with both hands. Try to take five deep breaths.

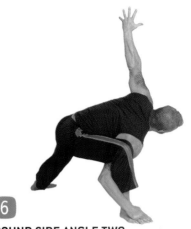

6

BOUND SIDE ANGLE TWO

Inhale, keep your right hand wrapped around that ankle, and raise your left arm to the sky. Stay here if you must, or move to Bound Side Angle Three.

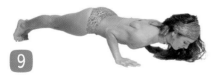

9

LOWER DOWN

Lower your body down slowly 3 . . . 2 . . . 1 while you squeeze your elbows in toward your ribs, making sure that your shoulders don't dip below your elbows. Now hover three inches off the mat, if possible, and hold for a count of 3 . . . 2 . . . 1. Then fully exhale and lower yourself to the mat.

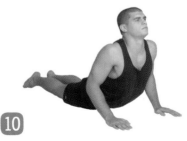

10

COBRA

Inhale, lengthen into Cobra, press your palms into the floor, lift your chest, roll your shoulders back, and look up.

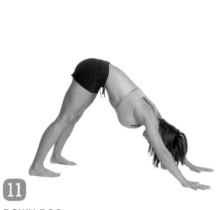

11

DOWN DOG

Exhale and push back into Down Dog by lifting your hips and pushing your chest back toward your feet while you take two small steps forward.

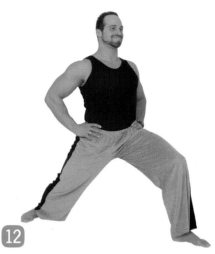

12

LEFT LUNGE HANDS ON HIPS

Inhale, sweep your left foot into a forward lunge, and place your right foot flat.

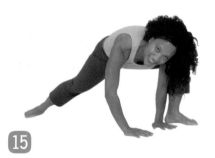

15

LOW LUNGE

Exhale as you drop down and bring your hands to the inside of your left foot.

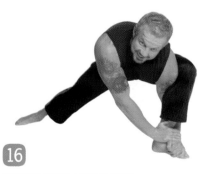

16

BOUND SIDE ANGLE ONE

Move your left arm beneath your left knee. See if you can grab your left ankle with both hands. Try to take five deep breaths.

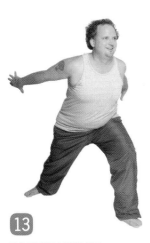

13

POSITION THREE

On your next inhalation, swing your arms back behind you and take flight again.

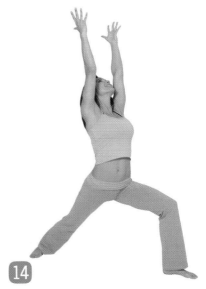

14

WARRIOR ONE

Inhale and reach your arms to the sky, squeeze your shoulders back, lift your chest, and look up at your hands in Warrior One.

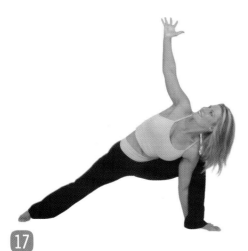

17

BOUND SIDE ANGLE TWO

Inhale, keep your left hand wrapped around your ankle, and raise your right arm to the sky. Stay here if you must, or move to Bound Side Angle Three.

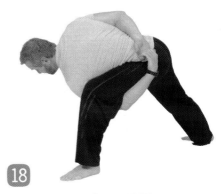

18

BOUND SIDE ANGLE THREE

Exhale, drop your right hand behind your back, and clasp those hands together in Bound Side Angle. Now inhale, squeeze your shoulder blades toward each other, keep those hands clasped behind you, and try to lean your head back. Try to take four more deep breaths.

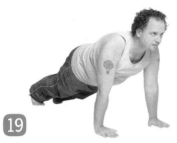

19 PUSH-UP POSITION

Lower your hands to the mat, and step or jump back into a push-up position.

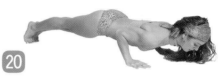

20 LOWER DOWN

Lower your body down slowly 3 . . . 2 . . . 1 while you squeeze your elbows in toward your ribs, making sure that your shoulders don't dip below your elbows. Now hover three inches off the mat, if possible, and hold for a count of 3 . . . 2 . . . 1. Then fully exhale and lower yourself to the mat.

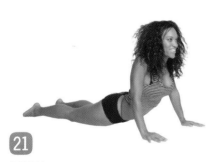

21 COBRA

Inhale, lengthen into Cobra, press your palms into the floor, lift your chest, roll your shoulders back, and look up.

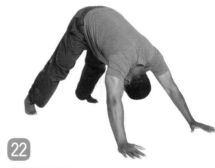

22 DOWN DOG

Exhale and push back into Down Dog by lifting your hips and pushing your chest back toward your feet while you take two small steps forward.

OPEN YOUR CAN AND WALK THE PLANK

This sequence has the **Can Opener** position, which is the mack daddy of hip openers. It opens and stretches your glutes, illiotibial (IT) bands, and the muscles of the lower back. Can Opener is like a pressure-washer for your hips, pelvis, and low back. It blasts away built-up tension in these areas and resets you for the tasks at hand. Remember to be patient with this one. You don't need to have your chest on the floor in order to receive its benefits. If you're breathing deeply and feeling a deep stretch in your hips, you're doing great! I will always do this position before I get in the ring; it has saved me countless times.

As Yoga-Doc can confirm, Can Opener opens all of the gluteal muscles, the IT bands, the pyriformis muscles, and the muscles of the lower back. Just be careful not to push too hard on this one, or your knees might take on too much torquing stress.

We've also included the **Side Plank** for pure shoulder, leg, and core strength. We cut this position up into three steps, so do what you can and keep working toward Position Three. But take your time. You'll master this one sooner than you think.

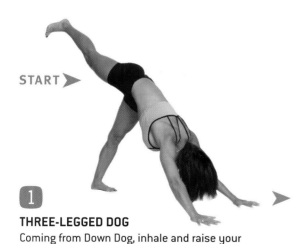

START ▶

1

THREE-LEGGED DOG
Coming from Down Dog, inhale and raise your right leg high.

2

CAN OPENER PREP
Exhale and lunge forward with your right leg. Draw your bent right knee behind your right hand and drop the leg down. Drop your left knee to the ground and lower down onto your right glute.

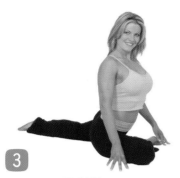

3

CAN OPENER ONE

Inhale, lift your chest, roll your shoulders back, and look up as you press into the ground.

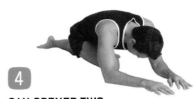

4

CAN OPENER TWO

Exhale, reach your arms forward, and see if you can sink deeper. Take four deep breaths as you press your left hip forward and your right hip down and back.

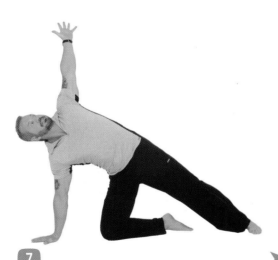

7

RIGHT SIDE PLANK ONE

Now, drop that right knee to the ground, bring your right hand directly underneath your right shoulder, and reach your left arm to the sky.

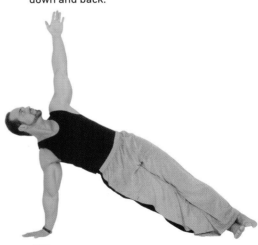

8

RIGHT SIDE PLANK TWO

If you can, straighten your right leg, pull your core in toward your spine, and push your hips toward the sky as your press into that right hand.

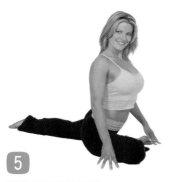

➤ **5**

CAN OPENER ONE

Inhale, lift your chest, and roll your shoulders back as you return once more to Can Opener One.

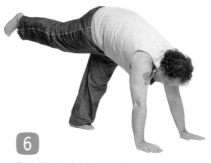

➤ **6**

THREE-LEGGED DOG

Exhale, curl the toes of your left foot, and push back through Down Dog. Raise that right leg high. Shake it like a dog.

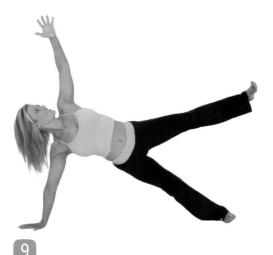

➤ **9**

RIGHT SIDE PLANK THREE

Now, try to raise your left leg up toward the sky.

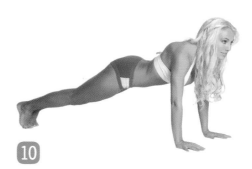

➤ **10**

PUSH-UP POSITION

Exhale, drop your hands and left foot back to the mat, and step back into a push-up position.

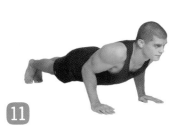

11

LOWER DOWN

Lower your body down slowly 3 . . . 2 . . . 1 as you squeeze your elbows in toward your ribs, making sure that your shoulders don't dip below your elbows. Now hover three inches off the mat if possible, and hold 3 . . . 2 . . . 1. Then exhale, and lower yourself to the mat.

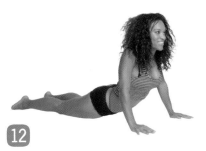

12

COBRA

Inhale and lengthen into Cobra.

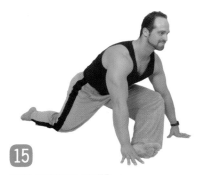

15

CAN OPENER PREP

Exhale and lunge forward with your left leg. Draw your bent left knee behind your left hand and drop the leg down. Drop your right knee to the ground and lower down onto your left glute.

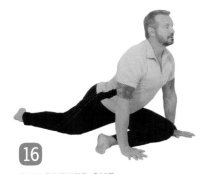

16

CAN OPENER ONE

Inhale, lift your chest, roll your shoulders back, and look up as you press your palms into the ground.

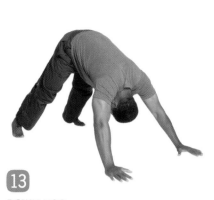

➤ **13**

DOWN DOG
Exhale and push back into Down Dog.

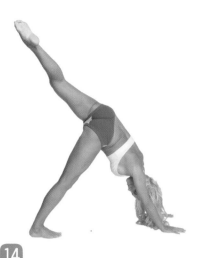

➤ **14**

THREE-LEGGED DOG
Inhale and raise your left leg high.

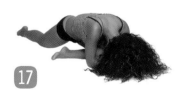

➤ **17**

CAN OPENER TWO
Exhale, reach your arms forward, and see if you can sink deeper. Take four deep breaths as you press your right hip forward and your left hip down and back.

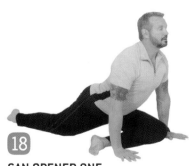

➤ **18**

CAN OPENER ONE
Inhale, lift your chest, and roll your shoulders back.

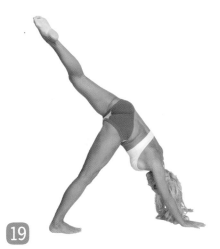

19

THREE-LEGGED DOG

Exhale, curl the toes of your right foot, and push back through Down Dog and raise that left leg high. Shake it like a dog.

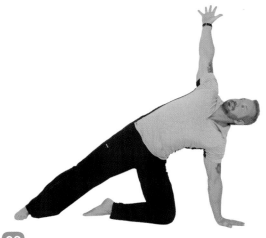

20

LEFT SIDE PLANK ONE

Now, drop that left knee to the ground, bring your left hand directly underneath your left shoulder, and reach your right arm to the sky.

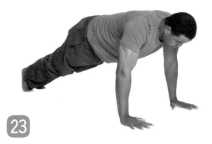

23

PUSH-UP POSITION

Exhale, drop your hands and right foot to the mat, and step back into a push-up position.

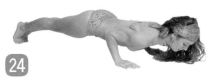

24

LOWER DOWN

Lower your body down slowly 3 . . . 2 . . . 1 as you squeeze your elbows in toward your ribs, making sure that your shoulders don't dip below your elbows. Now hover three inches off the mat if possible, and hold 3 . . . 2 . . . 1. Then exhale, and lower yourself to the mat.

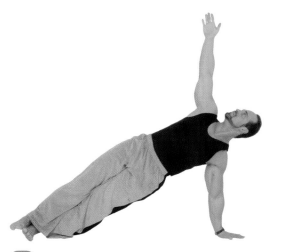

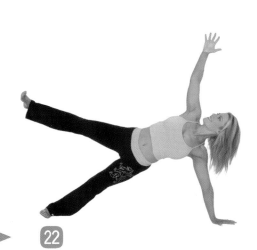

➤ **21**

LEFT SIDE PLANK TWO
If you can, straighten your left leg, pull your core in toward your spine, and push your hips toward the sky as your press into that left hand.

➤ **22**

LEFT SIDE PLANK THREE
Now try to raise your right leg up toward the sky.

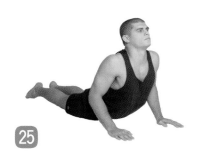

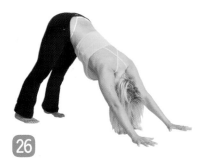

➤ **25**

COBRA
Inhale and lengthen into Cobra.

➤ **26**

DOWN DOG
Exhale and push back into Down Dog. Take a deep inhalation.

> **HOT TIP!**
> If you have shoulder problems, Side Plank is your answer. The longer you stay in this position, the stronger your shoulders will become.

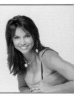

YRG WORKOUTS AT A GLANCE

Check out pages 120 to 129 once you know the YRG lay of the land and just want to get a 20-Minute Workout without all of the explanations. You can use it as a quick-reference road map anywhere, anytime. If you want a longer, more challenging workout, insert the 30-Minute (pages 130–133) and 45-Minute (pages 134–141) add-ons and substitutions for the newer positions from the 30- and 45-Minute Workouts.

IGNITION

FIRE UP THE BACK AND HIPS

TOUCHDOWNS AND SIDE BENDS

RAINING CATS, DOGS, AND COBRAS

BROKEN TABLE, BROKEN TABLE PLUS OR FIX THE BROKEN TABLE

GET HOT

WINGS AND THINGS

MEET THE WARRIOR

+SWEAT YOUR ASS OFF OR SWEAT YOUR ASS OFF AND TWIST

+RUSSIAN LEG SWEEPS

+WRAP AND BURN

+OPEN YOUR CAN AND WALK THE PLANK

BRING IT ON HOME

GO HOME

THE FINISH

➤ IGNITION

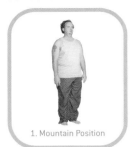
1. Mountain Position

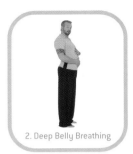
2. Deep Belly Breathing

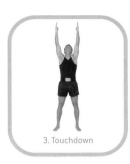
3. Touchdown

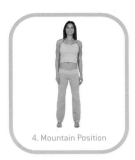
4. Mountain Position

➤ FIRE UP THE BACK AND HIPS

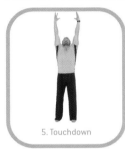
5. Touchdown

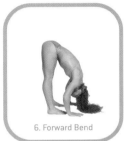
6. Forward Bend

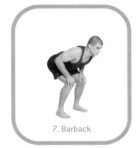
7. Barback

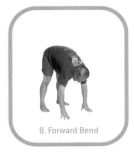
8. Forward Bend

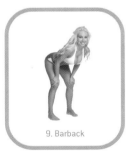
9. Barback

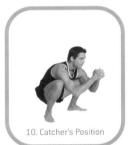
10. Catcher's Position

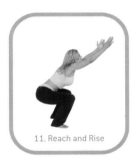
11. Reach and Rise

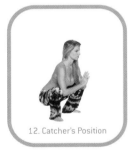
12. Catcher's Position

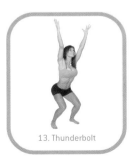
13. Thunderbolt

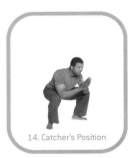
14. Catcher's Position

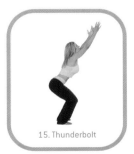
15. Thunderbolt

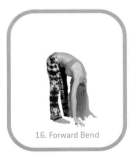
16. Forward Bend

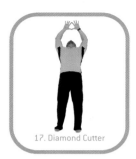

17. Diamond Cutter

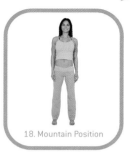

18. Mountain Position

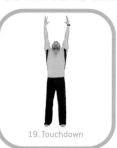

19. Touchdown

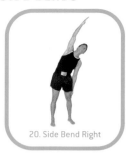

20. Side Bend Right

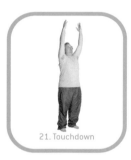

21. Touchdown

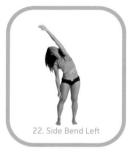

22. Side Bend Left

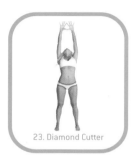

23. Diamond Cutter

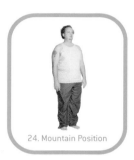

24. Mountain Position

➤ RAINING CATS, DOGS, AND COBRAS

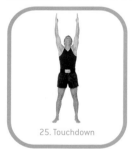

25. Touchdown

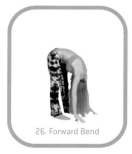

26. Forward Bend

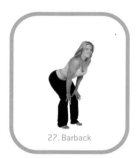

27. Barback

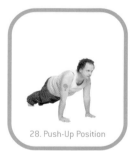

28. Push-Up Position

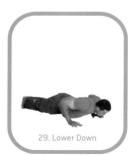

29. Lower Down

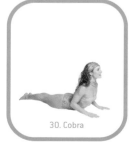

30. Cobra

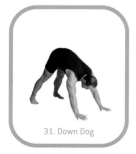

31. Down Dog

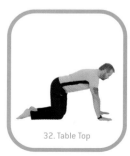

32. Table Top

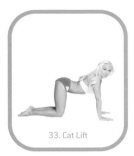

33. Cat Lift

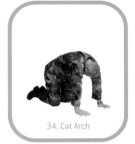

34. Cat Arch

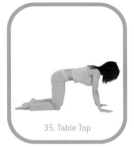

35. Table Top

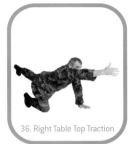

36. Right Table Top Traction

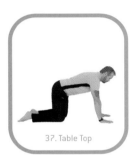

37. Table Top

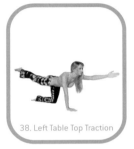

38. Left Table Top Traction

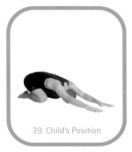

39. Child's Position

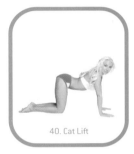

40. Cat Lift

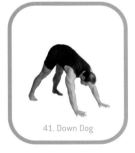

41. Down Dog

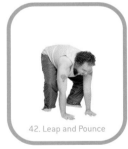

42. Leap and Pounce

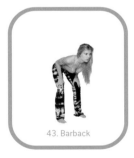

43. Barback

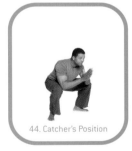

44. Catcher's Position

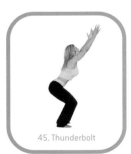

45. Thunderbolt

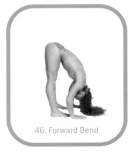

46. Forward Bend

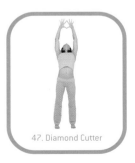

47. Diamond Cutter

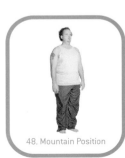

48. Mountain Position

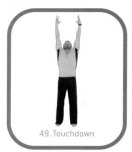

49. Touchdown

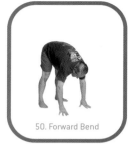

50. Forward Bend

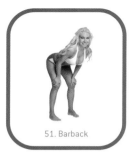

51. Barback

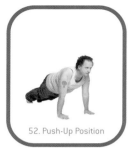

52. Push-Up Position

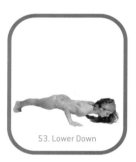

53. Lower Down

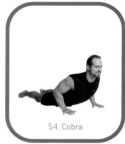

54. Cobra

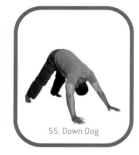

55. Down Dog

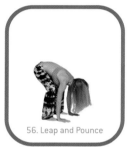

56. Leap and Pounce

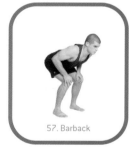

57. Barback

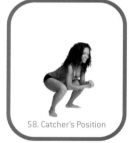

58. Catcher's Position

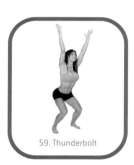

59. Thunderbolt

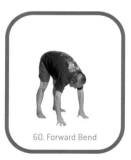

60. Forward Bend

➤ WINGS AND THINGS

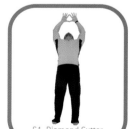

61. Diamond Cutter

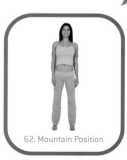

62. Mountain Position

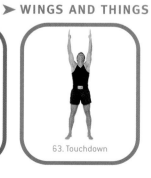

63. Touchdown

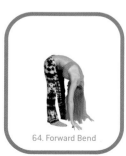

64. Forward Bend

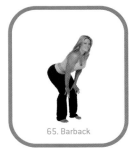
65. Barback

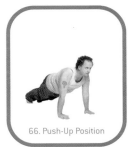
66. Push-Up Position

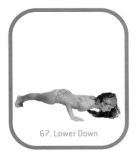
67. Lower Down

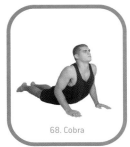
68. Cobra

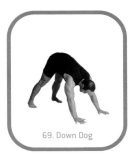
69. Down Dog

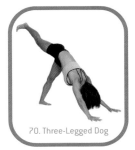
70. Three-Legged Dog

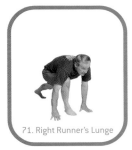
71. Right Runner's Lunge

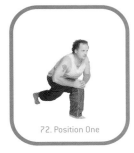
72. Position One

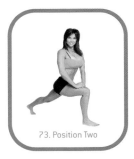
73. Position Two

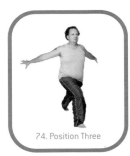
74. Position Three

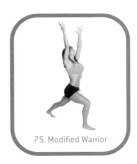
75. Modified Warrior

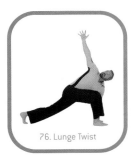
76. Lunge Twist

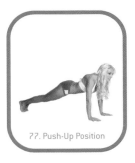
77. Push-Up Position

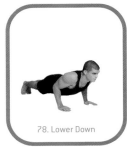
78. Lower Down

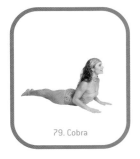
79. Cobra

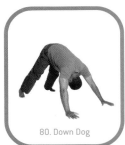
80. Down Dog

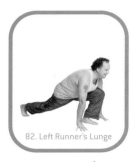
81. Three-Legged Dog

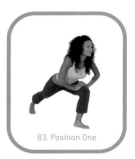
82. Left Runner's Lunge

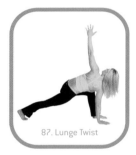
83. Position One

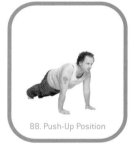
84. Position Two

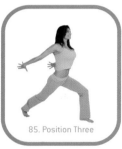
85. Position Three

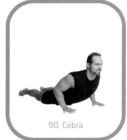
86. Modified Warrior

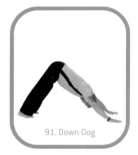
87. Lunge Twist

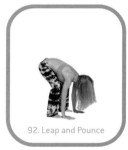
88. Push-Up Position

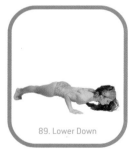
89. Lower Down

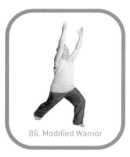
90. Cobra

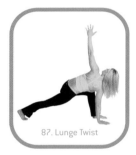
91. Down Dog

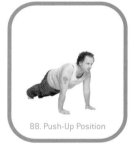
92. Leap and Pounce

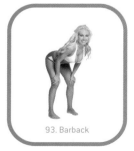
93. Barback

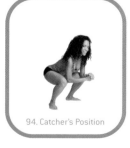
94. Catcher's Position

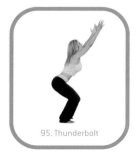
95. Thunderbolt

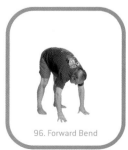
96. Forward Bend

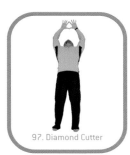

97. Diamond Cutter

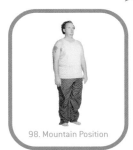

98. Mountain Position

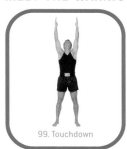

99. Touchdown

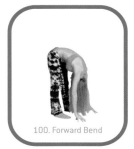

100. Forward Bend

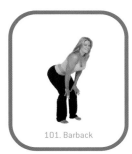

101. Barback

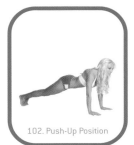

102. Push-Up Position

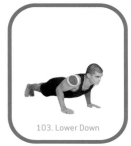

103. Lower Down

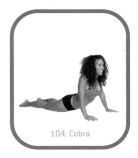

104. Cobra

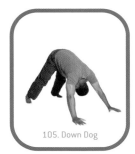

105. Down Dog

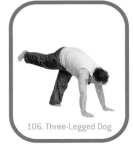

106. Three-Legged Dog

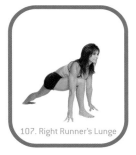

107. Right Runner's Lunge

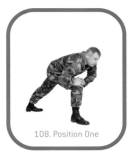

108. Position One

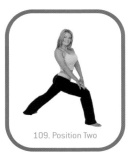

109. Position Two

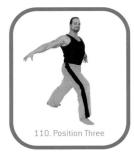

110. Position Three

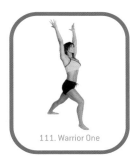

111. Warrior One

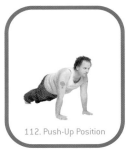

112. Push-Up Position

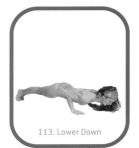

113. Lower Down

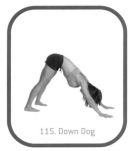

114. Cobra

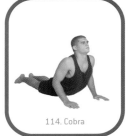

115. Down Dog

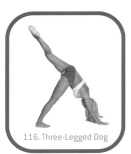

116. Three-Legged Dog

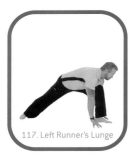

117. Left Runner's Lunge

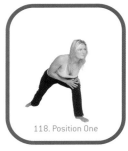

118. Position One

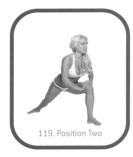

119. Position Two

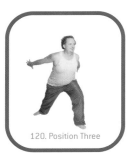

120. Position Three

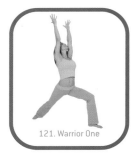

121. Warrior One

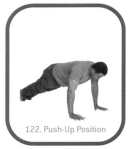

122. Push-Up Position

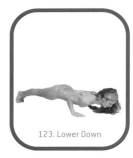

123. Lower Down

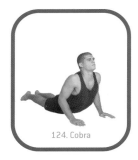

124. Cobra

> **BRING IT ON HOME**

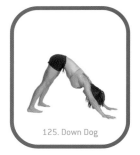

125. Down Dog

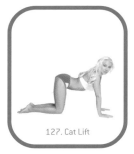

126. Table Top

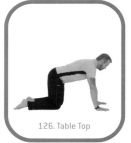

127. Cat Lift

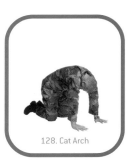

128. Cat Arch

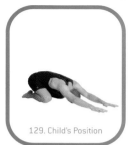

129. Child's Position

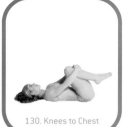

130. Knees to Chest

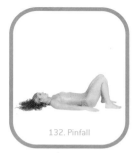

131. Dead Bug

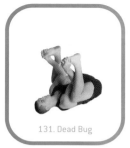

132. Pinfall

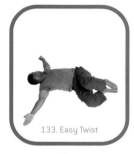

133. Easy Twist

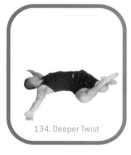

134. Deeper Twist

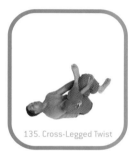

135. Cross-Legged Twist

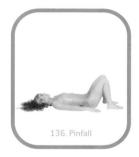

136. Pinfall

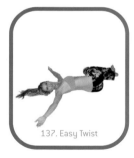

137. Easy Twist

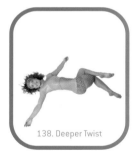

138. Deeper Twist

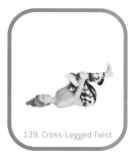

139. Cross-Legged Twist

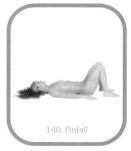

140. Pinfall

➤ **THE FINISH**

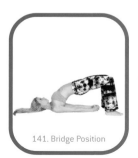

141. Bridge Position

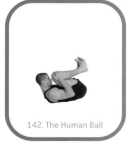

142. The Human Ball

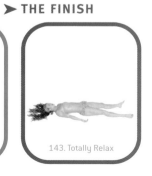

143. Totally Relax

➤ **BROKEN TABLE PLUS** *Substitute this for Broken Table*

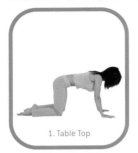
1. Table Top

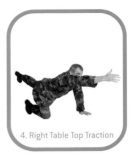
2. Right Table Top Traction

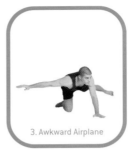
3. Awkward Airplane

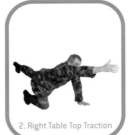
4. Right Table Top Traction

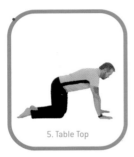
5. Table Top

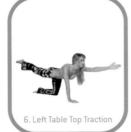
6. Left Table Top Traction

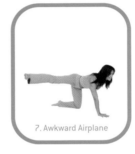
7. Awkward Airplane

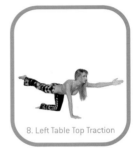
8. Left Table Top Traction

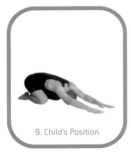
9. Child's Position

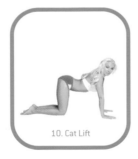
10. Cat Lift

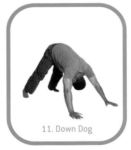
11. Down Dog

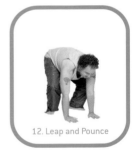
12. Leap and Pounce

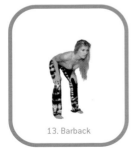
13. Barback

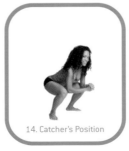
14. Catcher's Position

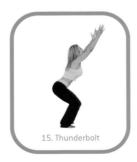
15. Thunderbolt

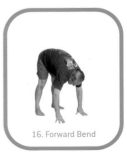
16. Forward Bend

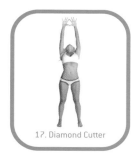

17. Diamond Cutter

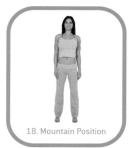

18. Mountain Position

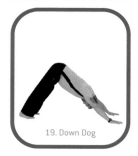

19. Down Dog

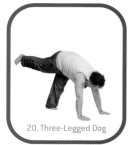

20. Three-Legged Dog

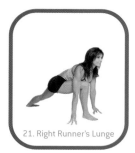

21. Right Runner's Lunge

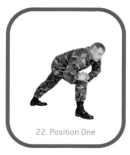

22. Position One

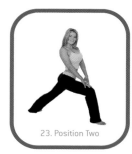

23. Position Two

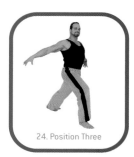

24. Position Three

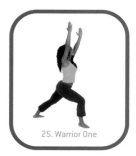

25. Warrior One

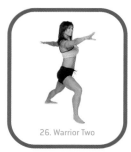

26. Warrior Two

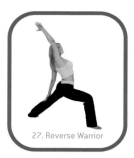

27. Reverse Warrior

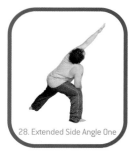

28. Extended Side Angle One

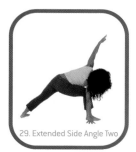

29. Extended Side Angle Two

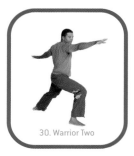

30. Warrior Two

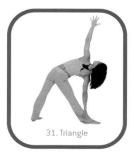

31. Triangle

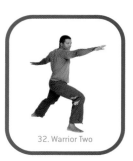

32. Warrior Two

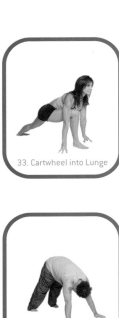

33. Cartwheel into Lunge

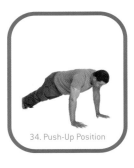

34. Push-Up Position

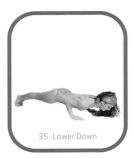

35. Lower Down

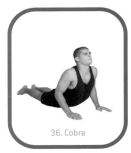

36. Cobra

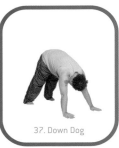

37. Down Dog

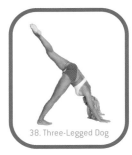

38. Three-Legged Dog

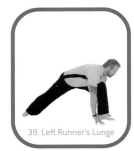

39. Left Runner's Lunge

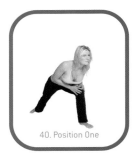

40. Position One

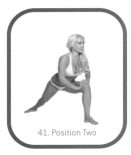

41. Position Two

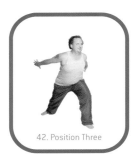

42. Position Three

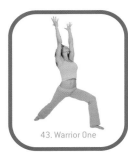

43. Warrior One

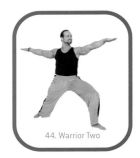

44. Warrior Two

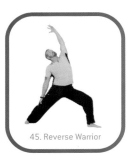

45. Reverse Warrior

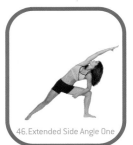

46. Extended Side Angle One

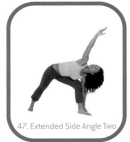

47. Extended Side Angle Two

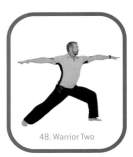

48. Warrior Two

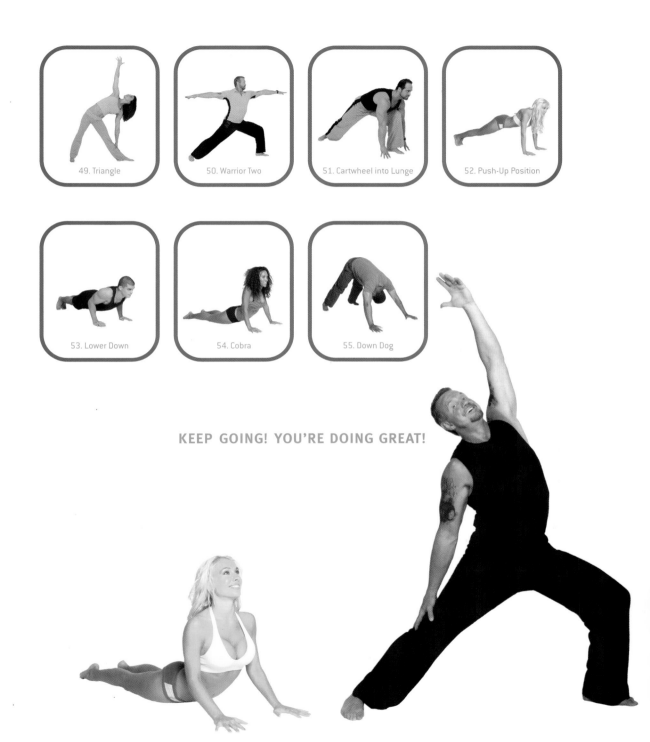

49. Triangle

50. Warrior Two

51. Cartwheel into Lunge

52. Push-Up Position

53. Lower Down

54. Cobra

55. Down Dog

KEEP GOING! YOU'RE DOING GREAT!

➤ **FIX THE BROKEN TABLE** *Substitute this for Broken Table*

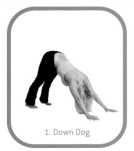

1. Down Dog

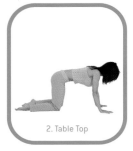

2. Table Top

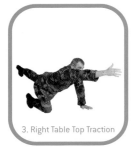

3. Right Table Top Traction

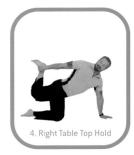

4. Right Table Top Hold

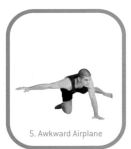

5. Awkward Airplane

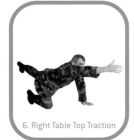

6. Right Table Top Traction

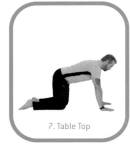

7. Table Top

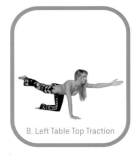

8. Left Table Top Traction

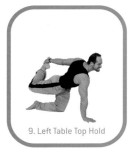

9. Left Table Top Hold

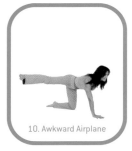

10. Awkward Airplane

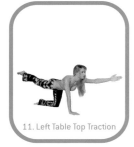

11. Left Table Top Traction

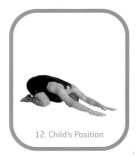

12. Child's Position

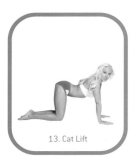

13. Cat Lift

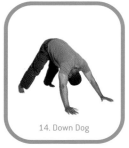

14. Down Dog

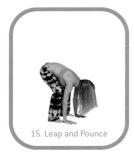

15. Leap and Pounce

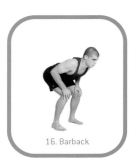

16. Barback

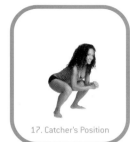

17. Catcher's Position

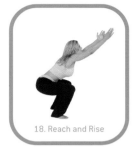

18. Reach and Rise

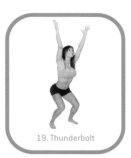

19. Thunderbolt

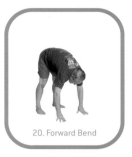

20. Forward Bend

+ SWEAT YOUR ASS OFF AND TWIST

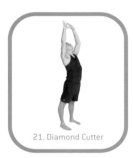

21. Diamond Cutter

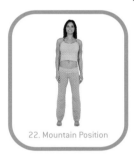

22. Mountain Position

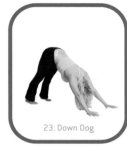

23. Down Dog

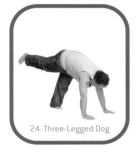

24. Three-Legged Dog

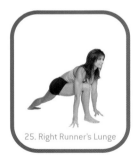

25. Right Runner's Lunge

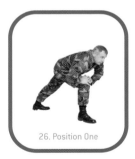

26. Position One

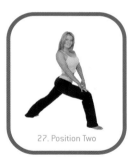

27. Position Two

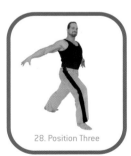

28. Position Three

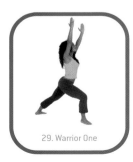

29. Warrior One

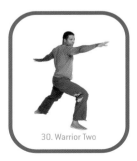

30. Warrior Two

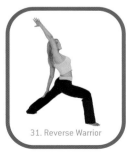

31. Reverse Warrior

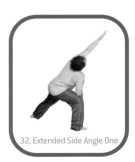

32. Extended Side Angle One

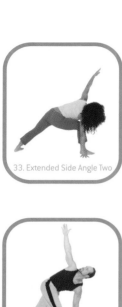

33. Extended Side Angle Two

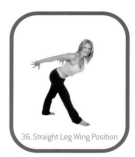

34. Warrior Two

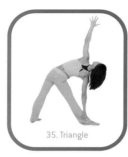

35. Triangle

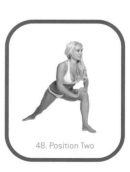

36. Straight Leg Wing Position

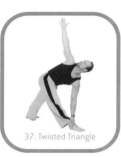

37. Twisted Triangle

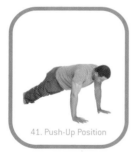

38. Straight Leg Wing Position

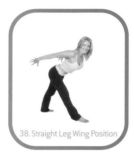

39. Warrior One

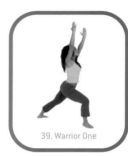

40. Right Runner's Lunge

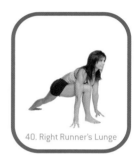

41. Push-Up Position

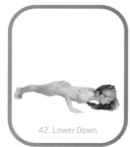

42. Lower Down

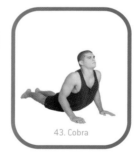

43. Cobra

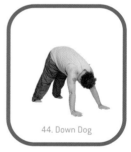

44. Down Dog

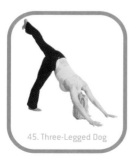

45. Three-Legged Dog

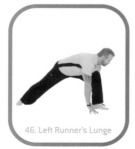

46. Left Runner's Lunge

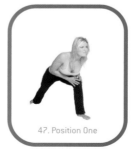

47. Position One

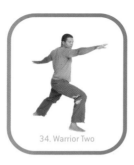

48. Position Two

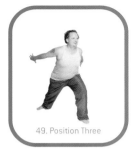

49. Position Three

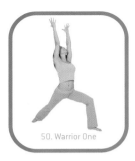

50. Warrior One

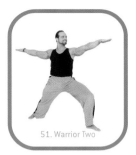

51. Warrior Two

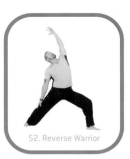

52. Reverse Warrior

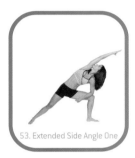

53. Extended Side Angle One

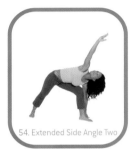

54. Extended Side Angle Two

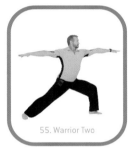

55. Warrior Two

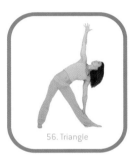

56. Triangle

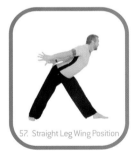

57. Straight Leg Wing Position

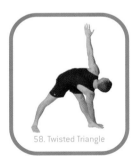

58. Twisted Triangle

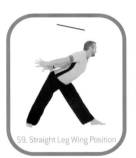

59. Straight Leg Wing Position

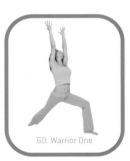

60. Warrior One

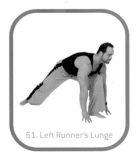

61. Left Runner's Lunge

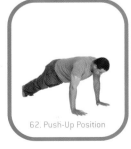

62. Push-Up Position

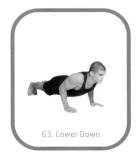

63. Lower Down

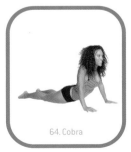

64. Cobra

+ RUSSIAN LEG SWEEPS

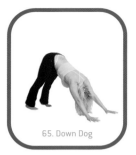

65. Down Dog

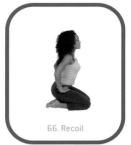

66. Recoil

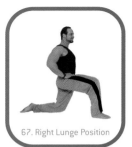

67. Right Lunge Position

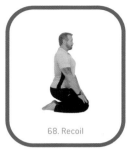

68. Recoil

+ WRAP AND BURN

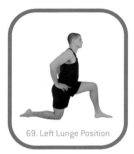

69. Left Lunge Position

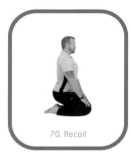

70. Recoil

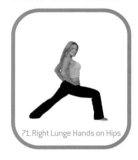

71. Right Lunge Hands on Hips

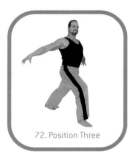

72. Position Three

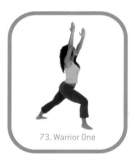

73. Warrior One

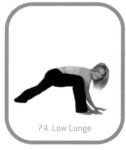

74. Low Lunge

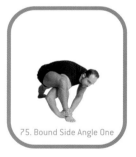

75. Bound Side Angle One

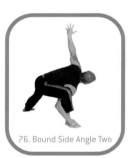

76. Bound Side Angle Two

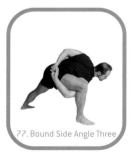

77. Bound Side Angle Three

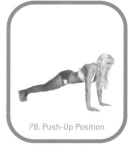

78. Push-Up Position

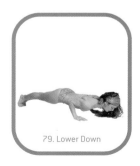

79. Lower Down

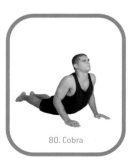

80. Cobra

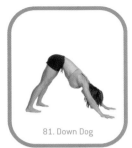
81. Down Dog

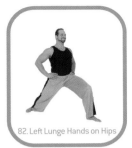
82. Left Lunge Hands on Hips

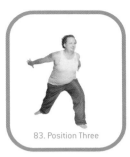
83. Position Three

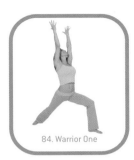
84. Warrior One

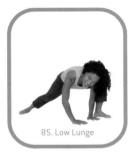
85. Low Lunge

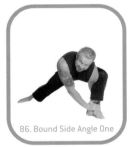
86. Bound Side Angle One

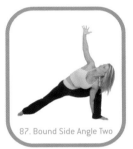
87. Bound Side Angle Two

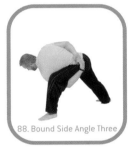
88. Bound Side Angle Three

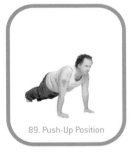
89. Push-Up Position

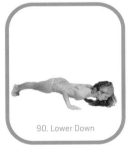
90. Lower Down

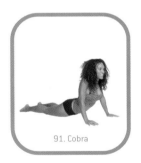
91. Cobra

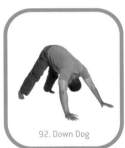
92. Down Dog

+ OPEN YOUR CAN AND WALK THE PLANK

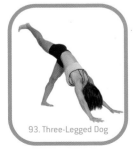
93. Three-Legged Dog

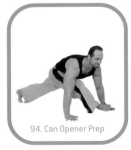
94. Can Opener Prep

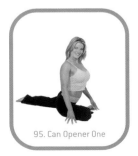
95. Can Opener One

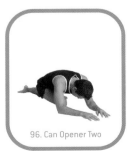
96. Can Opener Two

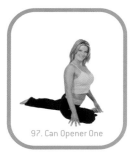

97. Can Opener One

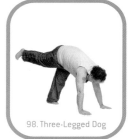

98. Three-Legged Dog

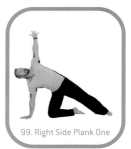

99. Right Side Plank One

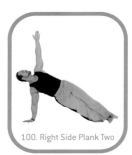

100. Right Side Plank Two

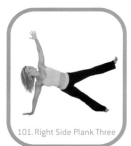

101. Right Side Plank Three

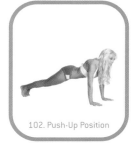

102. Push-Up Position

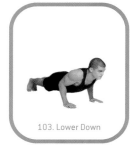

103. Lower Down

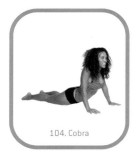

104. Cobra

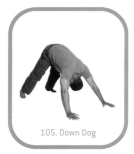

105. Down Dog

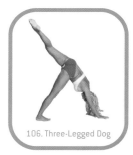

106. Three-Legged Dog

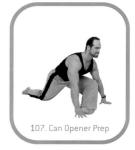

107. Can Opener Prep

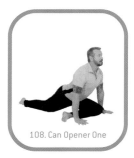

108. Can Opener One

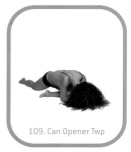

109. Can Opener Twp

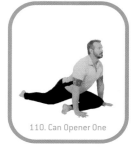

110. Can Opener One

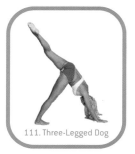

111. Three-Legged Dog

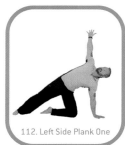

112. Left Side Plank One

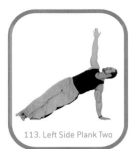
113. Left Side Plank Two

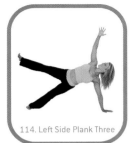
114. Left Side Plank Three

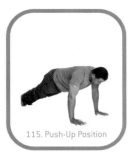
115. Push-Up Position

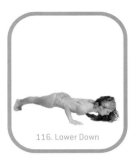
116. Lower Down

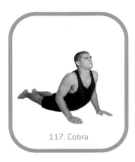
117. Cobra

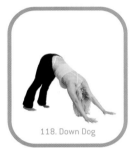
118. Down Dog

YOU DID IT!

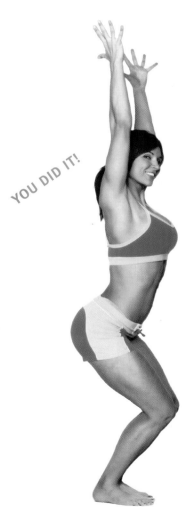

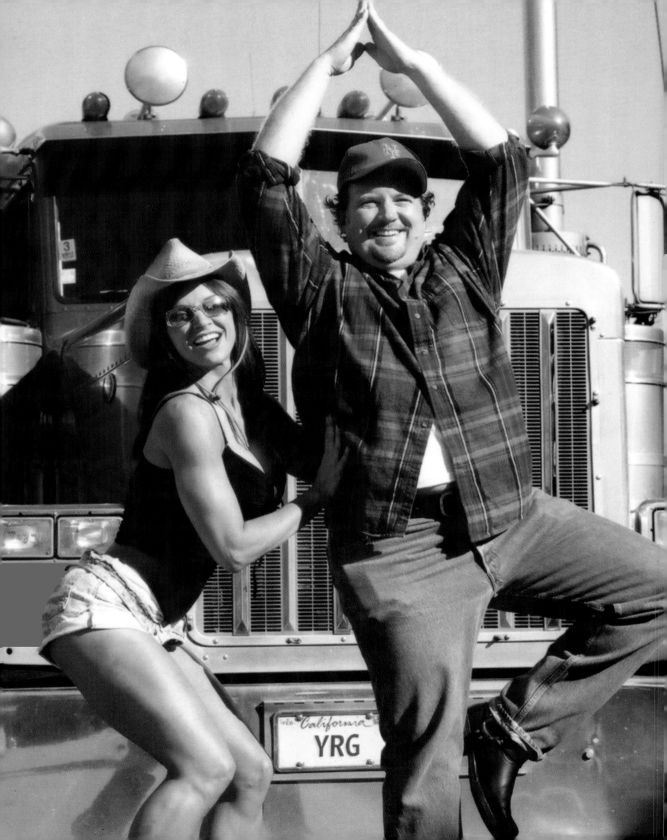

CHAPTER 3

HAMMERS AND DUCT TAPE

QUICK FIXES FOR INSTANT STRESS RELIEF

This chapter is a lot like Mom's chicken soup for a cold, ginger ale for an upset stomach, or a nice cold morning beer to chase away a hangover. "Hammers and Duct Tape" will provide you with some quick fixes and stop-gap measures for stress relief and joint rehabilitation. A lot of these exercises are old-school yoga positions, and some are positions I made up along the way to rehab and strengthen my body to help hold back the hands of time.

If you have problems in a particular area of your body, back, shoulders, knees, or hips and do these exercises, I'm telling you, you will increase the strength and flexibility in that area. The complete YRG workout is *the* perfect stress relief and rehab program for your entire body, but these stress busters and joint strengtheners are what you can use when you need to isolate a specific area of the body or if you are looking to build an arsenal of de-stress smart bombs to keep you cool and focused. These can all be performed in as short a period of time as three to five minutes for instant results. We even have a section on how to rev up your heart rate for a better cardio workout.

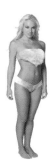

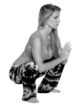

This little breathing exercise helps you calm your mind and relax your body in a minute or less! When you breathe this way, you enable your body to fully utilize every bit of oxygen that you take in and pump it directly into your bloodstream for immediate use. Plus, you are expelling carbon dioxide (CO_2) and other waste products very efficiently on each exhalation. This is very similar to the technique on page 21, except you hold your breath on the inhalation.

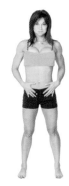

1 STAND UPRIGHT

Stand up in an upright position. You can also sit in a comfortable position on a chair or on the floor, or even lie on your back.

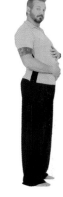

2 INHALE

Inhale through your nose gently and deeply, and slowly fill your lungs, then your stomach, full of air. Again: Your stomach, your belly, and your gut push out like Santa Claus as you pull all of that air deep into your lungs and then your stomach.

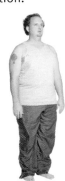

3 HOLD BREATH

Once you've filled your stomach full of air, hold the breath in for three counts without straining.

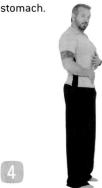

4 EXHALE

Then slowly exhale through your nose, controlling that exhalation until every last bit of CO_2 leaves your body. As you are doing this, pull your stomach toward your rib cage to help push the air out. Now inhale once again.

Repeat the cycle five more times and feel the buzz!

Camel to Child's Position: Great Posture and Back Strengthener

Camel is a strong extension, while **Child's Position** is an easy flexion, which will help you knock the rust off that steel spine so you can be more pliable, open, and relaxed. It works! You can take it from us—or from the Tibetan monks who typically live well into their eighties. Camel opens your chest, shoulders, and neck, while it stabilizes and strengthens your abs, quads, pelvis, and back. After you hold Camel for three to five breaths, you counter-pose with Child's Position in order to create internal and musculo-skeletal balance.

> **YOGA-DOC SAYS . . .**
> This sequence originally comes from a program called the Tibetan Five Rites, which was used by monks each morning for the maintenance of general health and longevity. It starts with Camel, which is a great extension posture and back strengthener. The Camel pose counteracts the slumping forward and caving inward postural distortion that we all fall into when sitting at a desk, driving, or flying for many hours at a time.

1 CAMEL PREP
Kneel on your mat with your knees hip-width apart and your ass off of your knees. Curl your toes under, or if you're more flexible, keep the tops of your feet on the floor.

2 HALF CAMEL
Press your hips forward and squeeze your belly in while leaning your upper body back.

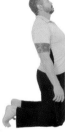

3 FULL CAMEL
Reach back and grab your heels while lifting your chest and squeezing your shoulder blades toward your spine. Lean your head all the way back, if you can, and hold for three to five breaths.

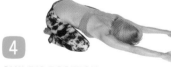

4 CHILD'S POSITION
Now fold into Child's Position by dropping your ass back to your heels while reaching your arms forward and resting your head on the mat.

Repeat this entire sequence five to seven times.

This yoga move is named the **Fish** because when you are in this position, your body resembles the spine of a fish—not because you'll get bug eyes and large-mouth bass lips if you stay in the position too long. Fish is similar to Camel because it is a great extension posture, which opens the chest, shoulders, and neck. The Fish was designed for you to be able to stay in the position for three to ten minutes at a time. If you tried to hold the Camel Position for this long, you would probably think that you were about to jettison a testicle around halfway through.

Start out slow and do Fish for about three minutes, and then work your way to extending the time if you can. Use supportive pillows or rolled-up blankets under your spine for both support and comfort when you shoot for five minutes or more. Fish posture will really relax the stress you have been carrying all week long.

YOGA-DOC SAYS . . .

The Fish is the one position I teach to every patient in my office who comes in with the forward head carry, a.k.a. the "turtle neck," or for those who have lost their normal cervical curve due to car accidents, falls, sports injuries, or just plain, old-fashioned sit-on-your-ass-too-long-itis! Recent studies say that we need to hold the neck and shoulders in a position like the Fish for up to ten minutes or more every day in order to effectively correct the forward head carry postural distortion. It should be performed on a daily basis until the optimal level of postural correction is achieved.

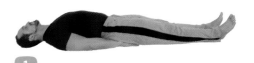

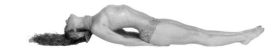

1

LIE DOWN
Lie on your back and place your hands, palms down, under your glutes.

2

FISH
Now lean into your elbows and lift your chest and head up off of the floor. Squeeze your shoulder blades toward each other, straighten your legs, and lean your head back.

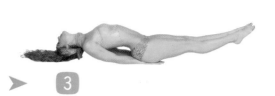

➤

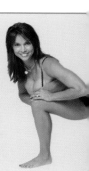

➤

HOT TIP!

Don't worry if the crown of your head does not touch the floor. Just keep leaning back and squeezing it all together. If you would like to let the crown of your head touch the floor, just slide your hands down toward your feet a few inches. If your crown does touch the mat, press it into the floor while lifting your chest.

3

AB WORK

If you want to add some ab work, lift your straight legs slowly up and down for a ten count or try to keep them raised for a ten count. This will burn your abs and strengthen your core while you traction your neck.

Thunderbolt to Forward Bend: Strengthen Your Core and Raise Your Heart Rate

This is another easy sequence that can both raise your heart rate as well as release low back, shoulder, and neck tension in a New York minute. **Thunderbolt** strengthens and stabilizes you from head to toe. It's all about engaging and flexing each muscle to your bones and watching your breath. Repeat this sequence five times. As you do Thunderbolt, it's important to inhale on the way up and exhale on the way down; it will definitely raise your heart rate.

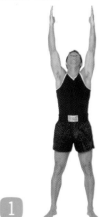

➤

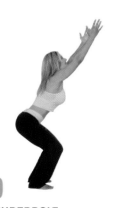

➤

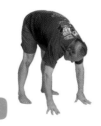

1

TOUCHDOWN

Stand with your feet hip-width apart. Inhale and reach your arms up into Touchdown.

2

THUNDERBOLT

Exhale and slowly squat until your thighs are parallel to the floor. Lift your chest, squeeze your shoulder blades back, and look up for one to three deep breaths.

3

FORWARD BEND

Exhale, straighten your legs, and lean into the pose for one to three deep breaths.

Repeat this sequence five times.

Shoulder Stand: Mother of All Yoga Postures

Shoulder Stand is not the easiest position for the Regular Guy to just pop up into, but do the best you can. You can receive many health benefits by simply lying on your back and placing your legs up the wall. You can work yourself into the full Shoulder Stand position in good time.

YOGA-DOC SAYS . . .

The **Shoulder Stand** is called the "mother of all yoga postures" because of its many health benefits. It has been reported to help balance the thyroid and parathyroid glands. It helps to gently recirculate tired veinous blood back to the heart while also helping to reset the lymphatic system. Shoulder Stand is said to calm the nervous system, which can help with insomnia, colds, headaches, asthma, and digestive difficulties.

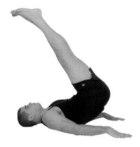

1

LEGS UP
Lie on your back and raise your legs and hips off the floor and up toward the ceiling.

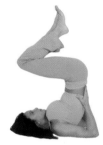

2

ELBOW PROP-UP
Place your hips in your hands, with your elbows placed firmly onto the floor. Press the back of your head onto the floor and lift your chin slightly to activate your neck muscles and stabilize your neck.

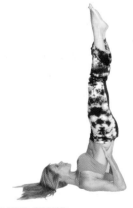

3

SHOULDER STAND
Press your hands into the middle of your back for more spinal support. Only your head, shoulders, upper arms, and elbows touch the floor in this position. Breathe deeply and fully for ten to thirty deep breaths.

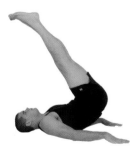

4

LOWER DOWN
When you are ready, place your hands back on the floor and slowly lower the back, hips, and legs to the floor. Rest for three to five deep breaths.

REHAB FOR BAD KNEES

When it comes to knee injuries and rehabilitation, I think I've been through it all. My first knee injury occurred at age twelve, after being hit by a car. The orthopedist said that the cartilage and ligament damage to my right knee was so extensive that I would never play football or hockey again. In fact, he warned that I would need a cane by age forty if I attempted to play any contact sports.

Since then, I've played a lot of contact sports, wrestled all over the world, injured both knees on many occasions, and learned a whole lot about how to strengthen and rehabilitate these old hinge joints. Oh, and by the way, I'm forty-eight years old, and as I'm writing this, about to make a comeback in the ring after a two-and-a-half-year layoff (knock on wood), I still don't need a cane! I deserve my money back for that bogus prognosis! These three suggested sequences help to strengthen and stretch the muscles that surround your knees. I've gotten back flexibility that they said was gone forever. Guess what? They were wrong.

YOGA-DOC SAYS . . .

These exercises are designed to create more flexibility, blood flow, and mechano-receptive nerve flow to the entire area. This allows for faster healing of the actual knee joint, as well as the knee's muscles of stabilization. If any of these exercises cause you a great deal of pain or discomfort, stop right away and consult a professional.

Russian Leg Sweeps: Knee Strengthener

This knee strengthener is the very same exercise you learned in the 45-Minute Workout. If at first you cannot do these leg sweeps, cheat 'til you don't have to cheat anymore. To build strength, you might have to push your hands on your thighs to help lift your ass off your heels. You might even have to use a chair at first to help get your ass off your heels. Do whatever it takes; you're building strength the entire time, and eventually you won't have to cheat.
See page 106 for the in-depth instructions.

Fire Up the Hips Sequence: Knee Strengthener

You are already familiar with this sequence from the second section of the 20-Minute Workout. I do this knee strengthener every day, sometimes twice. This exercise can be used as a warm up before physical activity or even when you're getting ready for work. It strengthens the low back along with all of the muscles that surround the hips and knees.
See pages 34–36 for a refresher on this knee-strengthening sequence.

Tiptoe Squats: This One Does It All!

Balancing exercises like this one cause the brain to connect with the rest of your body and help with your overall coordination. It's hard as hell when you first start, but when you get it, it's totally worth it. It speeds up the healing response by increasing blood flow and nerve flow while strengthening and stretching the lower body.

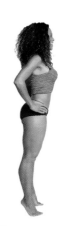

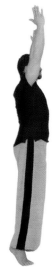

1

ON TIPTOES
Stand with your feet hip-width apart and get onto your tiptoes.

2

TIPTOE TOUCHDOWN
Now inhale and reach your arms up into Touchdown.

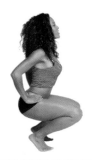

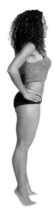

3

TIPTOE CATCHER'S POSITION
Exhale, and begin to squat down into Catcher's Position, keeping your hands on your hips, while on your toes for 5 . . . 4 . . . 3 . . . 2 . . . 1.

4

ON TIPTOES
Inhale, remain on your toes, and make your way back up to standing, for 5 . . . 4 . . . 3 . . . 2 . . . 1.

Repeat five times.

REHAB FOR TIGHT HIPS

Okay, guys, without these babies, DDP would never have wrestled well into his late forties. For starters, every single time I drop someone with the world-famous "Diamond Cutter," I land on my right hip—so needless to say, I have some seriously tight-ass hips. Without the exercises from this section of the book, I would be screwed. Now, if you sit on your ass all day, you're pretty much equally as screwed; your hip and back muscles will tighten and shorten. If you are a runner, a tennis player, or a hoops guy, then the continuous pounding on your hips also keeps you tighter than a drum. Stretching your hips can prevent injuries by keeping your lower body open and ready to deal with any physical challenges that your work, sports, or sex life might throw at you.

YOGA-DOC SAYS . . .

If you've ever sprained an ankle, injured a knee, or have flat feet, it is more than likely that your low back and hips have tightened in an attempt to stabilize and compensate for long-standing biomechanical insults, distortions, and scar tissue build-up that results from such injuries. In English, this means that your lower back and hip muscles can get very tight if you have injured your lower body or were born with bad knees or feet. It is immensely important to stretch the muscles that surround your hip joints in order to balance your pelvis and keep your weight evenly distributed between your back, hips, knees, ankles, and feet.

Crossed-Legged Stretch: Hip Opener

If you were ever backstage at a WWE, WCW, or TNA event, you would have seen me doing this hip opener right before they hit my music. It got my juices flowing and got my hips and knees ready for action. It can be done lying on your back or even sitting in a chair. It stretches the hip joint without putting much strain on the knee joint. You will also see me doing this exercise in the middle of meetings or anywhere I am sitting and starting to get stiff.

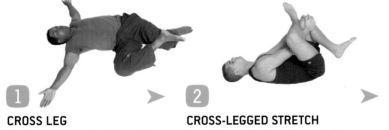

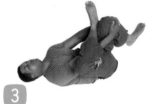

1 **CROSS LEG**
Lie down on your back or sit in a chair. Cross your right ankle just outside of your left knee.

2 **CROSS-LEGGED STRETCH**
Lean forward and grab your left knee with both hands. Pull your left knee back into your chest with both hands. Lean forward a bit more with each exhalation.

3 **DEEPER STRETCH**
Now lean back, roll your shoulders back, and pull your left knee back toward you a little more with each exhalation. Take seven to ten deep breaths.

Switch sides and repeat.

Dead Bug: Hip Opener

This is my favorite position of all. It's so easy, you can do it anywhere and any time of day, and it is a great hip opener that stretches your lower back and hips. Some people call it "Happy Baby," which also works for me since I feel like a happy baby when I'm in it. This pose looks funny as hell, but it really works your hips, lower back, and even your mid-back if you do it right. This is, without a doubt, one of my favorite positions.

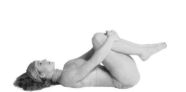 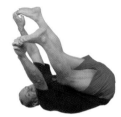 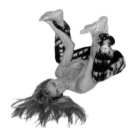

1

KNEES TO CHEST
Roll onto your back, pull your knees into your chest, and take three deep breaths.

2

DEAD BUG
Release your legs, let the soles of your feet face the sky, try to grab the outside of each foot, and pull the knees toward the ground.

3

FULL DEAD BUG
Roll your shoulders back and try to press your tailbone, your knees, and your head to the floor with each exhalation. Take seven to ten deep breaths.

I was taking a certain famous wrestler from San Antonio through this workout, who just happened to be a roommate of mine at the time. I won't name any names, but it sure is cold in here. You might even say it's Stone Cold. And as I told him to pull his knees toward the ground in Dead Bug, he looked at me and said, "I can't, kid. I'm afraid I'll shit myself!" So just in case you had one too many beers the night before you try this one, be careful here!

Can Opener: A Great Hip Opener

You guys probably remember this pressure washer for your hips, pelvis, and low back from the 45-Minute Workout. Remember to be patient with this one; you don't need to have your chest on the floor in order to receive the benefits from Can Opener. Just take it slow, breathe deeply, and feel the deep stretch!

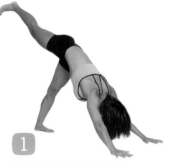

1

THREE-LEGGED DOG

From Down Dog, inhale and raise your right leg high.

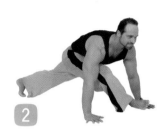

2

LUNGE AND LOWER DOWN

Exhale as your right leg lunges forward and slides over to your left wrist. Drop your left knee to the ground and lower down.

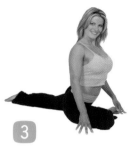

3

CAN OPENER ONE

Pull your right foot forward, moving to a 90-degree angle to increase this stretch, or you can pull that foot closer to your groin if you need to make it easier. Inhale, lift your chest, and roll your shoulders back.

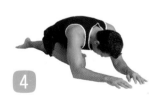

4

CAN OPENER TWO

Exhale, reach your arms forward, and sink deeper into Can Opener. Take seven to ten deep breaths.

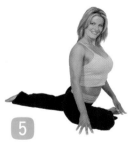

5

CAN OPENER ONE

Inhale, lift your chest, and roll your shoulders back.

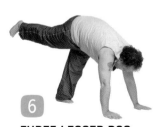

6

THREE-LEGGED DOG

Exhale, curl the toes of your left foot, push back through Down Dog, and raise that right leg high; shake it like a dog and move back to Down Dog.

Repeat, beginning with your left leg.

REHAB FOR BAD BACKS

Okay guys, who hasn't suffered some type of back injury or from a stiff or sore low back? Remember, I blew out a lumbar disc not long ago, and it was chiropractic kinesiology, massage, and yoga that got me back into action. The YRG workout is the perfect rehab program for your entire body, but check out these easy exercises when you are looking to keep your back healthy and strong.

YOGA-DOC SAYS . . .

These exercise sequences will help you keep it all together while your back is on the mend. We set up our rehab sequences in order to reset, balance, and stabilize the entire lower kinetic chain (feet, knees, hips, pelvis, and low back) for optimal function and peak performance.

Bring It on Home Sequence: Awaken the Spine

Okay, if we were doing one of our workouts, this sequence would mean we were almost done with the 20-Minute Workout. But like all of these sequences, it can be done all by its little lonesome, and I guarantee it will awaken your spine, get the blood flowing, and get you movin' right! *See page 66 to refresh your memory. Perform this sequence three to five times.*

Opposite Arm and Leg Traction with Broken Table: Spinal Rehab

If you want to rehab your spine, you are going to need the following: strengthening, stretching, balance, and traction. This exercise sequence has it all. In the beginning you're going to be tipping over like a teapot, but if you stick with it, your core will really start getting strong. This will also help to give you that tight ass you used to have; you can bounce a quarter off my ass, and by the time this book comes out I'll be fifty.

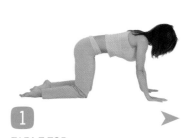

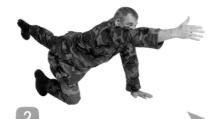

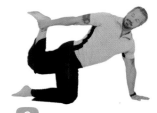

1

TABLE TOP
Move into Table Top.

2

RIGHT TABLE TOP TRACTION
Raise your left leg straight back and your right arm straight ahead. Reach and stretch. Take three deep breaths.

3

RIGHT TABLE TOP HOLD
Bend your left knee and grab your left ankle with your right hand. Take three deep breaths.

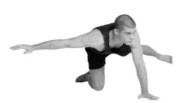

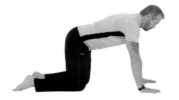

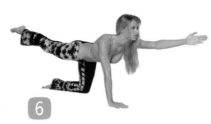

 4

AWKWARD AIRPLANE

Now straighten that leg and swing it to the left. As your right arm straightens to the right, reach and stretch. Take three deep breaths.

5

TABLE TOP

Exhale and drop back to Table Top.

6

LEFT TABLE TOP TRACTION

Raise your right leg straight back and your left arm straight ahead. Reach and stretch. Take three deep breaths.

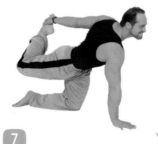

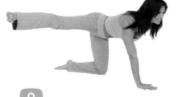

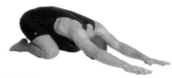

7

LEFT TABLE TOP HOLD

Bend your left knee and grab your left ankle with your right hand. Take three deep breaths.

8

AWKWARD AIRPLANE

Now straighten that leg and swing it to the right. As your left arm straightens to the left, reach and stretch. Take three deep breaths.

9

CHILD'S POSITION

Exhale and move to Child's Position. Take three deep breaths.

Go Home Sequence: Back Cool-Down

This one is a great post-workout cool-down, and that's why it appears at the end of the 20-Minute Sequence. It's also a perfect mini-workout because it stretches, bends, and wrings out all of your tense back muscles.

See pages 67–70 for in-depth instructions to this Back Rehab Sequence.

REHAB FOR SHOULDERS

Shoulder problems are common for anyone who has ever played football or tennis, thrown a baseball, or scrambled someone's brains with a steel chair. Whether you're swinging a hammer or swinging from the chandelier with your yoga-babe, your shoulders need to be strong, stable, and flexible. All of the slow-motion push-ups and shoulder openers in the YRG workout will give you what you need, but here are a few more yoga positions that will deliver the goods. Now remember, the shoulder is a complex joint, and if you are working with an injury, consult a professional to see which of these shoulder exercises suits you best.

Down Dog: All-in-One

YOGA-DOC SAYS . . .

Your dog does this position every morning upon waking. So let Fido teach you a new trick with this most efficient all-in-one position that strengthens your arms, opens your shoulders, relaxes your neck, and stretches your hamstrings and calves all at the same time!

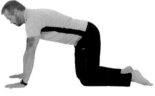

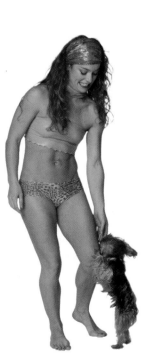

1 TABLE TOP

Start in Table Top with your hands and knees on the floor. Your shoulders should be directly over your hands, with your hips over your knees.

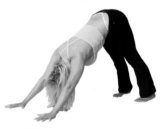

2 DOWN DOG

Now curl your toes, lift your ass to the ceiling, straighten your arms, press your chest back toward your legs, and take two small steps forward. Your neck is relaxed, your legs are as straight as possible, and your heels are pressing down toward the floor pigeon-toed. If your heels are nowhere near the floor, don't worry, because it all takes time. If you feel like your ass is about to scrape the ceiling, you're doing it right! Take five to seven deep breaths.

Repeat five times.

Side Plank: Stabilizer

You might remember this position from the end of the 45-Minute Workout. This position helps to stabilize and strengthen your wrists, shoulders, arms, and core. It's both a power and a balance position.

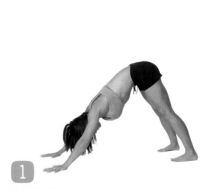

1 DOWN DOG
Begin in Down Dog. (You can even pick up from the Down Dog exercise on the previous page.)

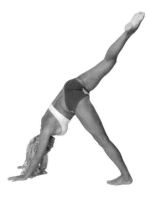

2 THREE-LEGGED DOG
Exhale, and push back through Three-Legged Dog. Raise that right leg high. Shake it like a dog.

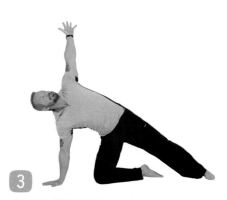

3 SIDE PLANK ONE
Now, drop that right knee to the floor while your left leg is stretched out toward the back of your mat and your left foot is flat. Straighten your right arm and make sure that your right hand is in direct alignment with your right shoulder. This will prevent shoulder injury. Now sweep your left hand to the sky and look up at your left hand, coming into Side Plank One. Hold this position for three to five deep breaths.

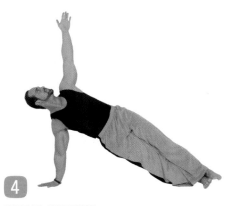

4 SIDE PLANK TWO
Now straighten that right leg so that both legs are together; keep pressing that right hand into the floor while you squeeze your belly in and lift your hips up toward the sky, coming into Side Plank Two. Hold this position for three to five deep breaths.

Now do the same sequence on the opposite side.

Shoulder Rolls: Opener

This one opens your shoulders and relaxes your neck while you stretch your back and hamstrings. When I first started this position, I was so tight I could barely even grab my hands, so I would use a towel to give myself a little cheat until I didn't have to cheat anymore. Today I can adjust my back just by grabbing my hands behind my back and rolling my shoulders back—I'm so glad I stuck with it.

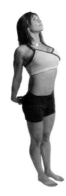

1

STAND TALL

Stand with your feet hip-width apart. Clasp your hands behind your back, interlace your fingers, and straighten your arms. Inhale, lift your chest and chin, and roll your shoulders back.

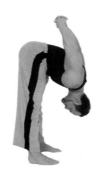

2

FOLD FORWARD

Exhale and fold forward as you pull those fists toward the ceiling, keep your legs straight, and relax your neck. Stay in this position for five deep breaths.

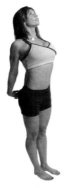

3

STAND TALL

Take a deep inhalation while you slowly come all the way up to standing, and lean way back.

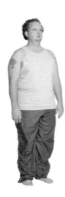

4

MOUNTAIN POSITION

Exhale, relax your arms to your sides, and let your body reset itself. It's easy to experience some dizziness while you're coming out of it, so do this one nice and slow.

HEART ACCELERATORS

Secrets to Increasing Your Heart Rate Fast

Try these heart accelerators when you want to rev up your heart rate. I do them all the time. Once you know what the hell you're doing, you can use them just about anywhere you want after you've warmed up in your YRG workout. They are guaranteed to awaken and energize your body and, of course, jack up your heart rate. Remember to always engage your muscles to your bones, like an isometric squeeze, while doing YRG, and especially these accelerators. *Please refer to Chapter 1, pages 23–26, "Ya Gotta Have Heart," for a refresher on finding your Maximum Aerobic Heart Rate.*

Bendin' Bolts

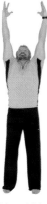

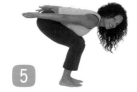

1

TOUCHDOWN
Stand with your feet hip-width apart. Inhale and reach your arms up into Touchdown.

2

THUNDERBOLT
Exhale and slowly squat until your thighs are parallel to the floor. Inhale, lift your chest, squeeze your shoulder blades back, and look up at your hands.

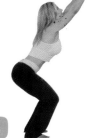

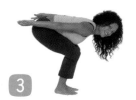

3

LIE FORWARD
Exhale, lay your nipples over your thighs, and sit back.

4

THUNDERBOLT
Inhale and lift your torso back up into Thunderbolt.

5

LIE FORWARD
Exhale, lean over your thighs, and sit back just a little lower.

Repeat the sequence until you reach your Maximum Aerobic Heart Rate.

Get hot as you rotate between Warrior One and Warrior Two.

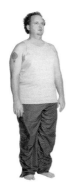

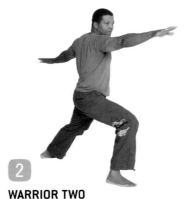

1

MOUNTAIN POSITION
Stand with your feet hip-width apart.

2

WARRIOR TWO
Now inhale, swing your right foot forward, and bend your right knee deeply as you bring your right arm forward and your left arm back. Exhale and strongly engage your arm and leg muscles to your bones.

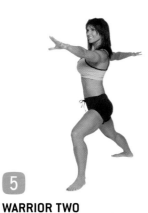

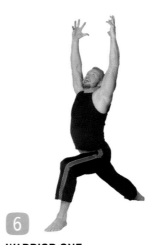

5

WARRIOR TWO
Exhale, move to Warrior Two by keeping that left knee bent, and bring your left arm forward and your right arm back as you look over that left hand.

6

WARRIOR ONE
Inhale and reach back up into Warrior One.

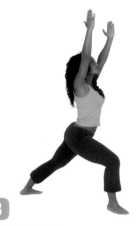

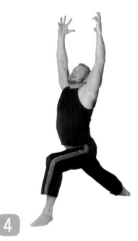

> **3**

WARRIOR ONE

Inhale and reach both arms to the sky as you lift your chest and roll your shoulder blades back into Warrior One.

> **4**

WARRIOR ONE

Exhale and pivot on the balls of your feet to rotate your whole body around so that you are facing the the back of your mat. Now your left knee is bending deeply.

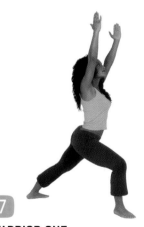

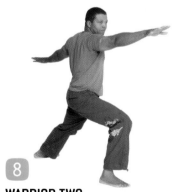

> **7**

WARRIOR ONE

Exhale, and rotate back to the front of your mat with your right knee bending deeply.

> **8**

WARRIOR TWO

Exhale, and move to Warrior Two once again.

Repeat steps 3 through 8 until you reach your Maximum Aerobic Heart Rate.

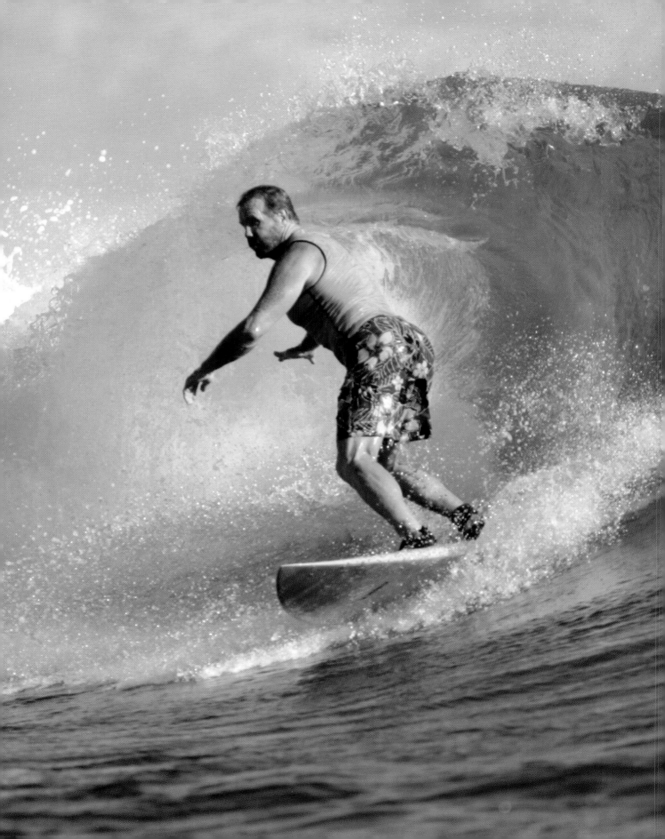

CHAPTER 4

DDP'S HEALTH TIPS AND PREVENTATIVE MAINTENANCE

In this chapter, Yoga-Doc and I will talk about ways to find what everyone is looking for: "The Fountain of Youth." We'll show you how to use *preventative maintenance* along with your yoga practice to keep your body at its peak level of performance, and give you guidelines for a healthy diet so you can lose weight, get healthy, find flexibility, and stay hard as long as possible. (You can let your mind drift here.) From icing your body, to organic juicing that supercharges your body and purifies your blood, to all kinds of different types of body repair work that I do in order to knock the bumps out after each of my matches, we'll give you the goods and tell you where to get ya some!

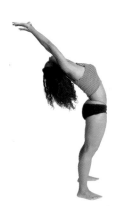
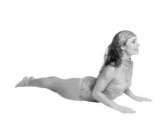
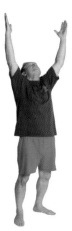

◄ Dallas finds the fountain of youth, surfing for the first time in twenty-seven years, all thanks to YRG.

HOLDING BACK THE HANDS OF TIME

Many people ask me how I managed to start my wrestling career at age thirty-five and stay at the top of my game well on my way to being fifty. As I am writing this book with the Yoga-Doc, I am once again on a comeback tour and back in the ring at the age of forty-eight. It's all about preventative maintenance and holding back the hands of time.

I have many friends in the wrestling business who could have lengthened their wrestling careers if they had just taken some extra time to fix the little problems before they turned into big ones. If these wrestlers just kept their bodies more finely tuned, like a NASCAR racer, they could be bouncing around in the squared circle long past their prime. I also know of some professional athletes who use some or all of the following healthy lifestyle tips, along with a serious yoga training program, and they've managed to beat the odds and prolong their careers way beyond expectation.

ICE vs. HEAT

How many times have you had an ache, pain, or injury and wondered whether you should use ice or heat on it? How many conflicting stories have you gotten from medical doctors, emergency room nurses, trainers, parents, or friends about the best post-training regimen? Is it ice only? Heat only? Ice for 15 minutes and then heat for 15 minutes? Moist heat or heating pad? Those questions are about as compelling as "What kind of mattress and pillow should I buy?" "Do you have a condom?" and "Hey, what's for dinner?"

Well, guys, don't worry, because we're here to give you all the best of our experience and expertise regarding this very confusing subject.

Icing Your Body

If you're an athlete, icing your body may be the most important habit you can adopt. The preventative maintenance starts by icing when you don't think you have to, like right after a hard workout or big game. This ritual can keep you from injuries *before* they happen and keep the swelling down, allowing your body to stay strong.

Fact: The NBA will not let any of its young players leave the arena until they have iced their knees, and some of these kids are only eighteen years old. Why? Because millions of dollars are wrapped up in these kids, and the NBA needs to protect its investments for them to pay off. The older players already understand that icing reduces swelling, which in turn reduces pain and injury.

Like most things in this world, icing is a pain in the ass, and it's hard to get yourself to do it unless you absolutely have to; but then again, if it was easy everyone would be doing it. It's *hard*, but it's the *hard* that makes it *great*. Most therapists say you should ice for 20 minutes, leave it off for 20, and then repeat. I personally will keep the ice on for 30 minutes or longer; then I switch to another area of my body. I call it the roaming ice bag.

When I first entered the world of professional wrestling, I was the first wrestler to ever ice my body. Believe it or not—the Boys (as we wrestlers call ourselves) would laugh and make jokes about me wrapping myself with ice bags. Stone Cold Steve Austin always had something to say to bust my balls (that SOB was always busting my balls—all in good fun). I remember one time Steve insisted that I strap a couple of Coors Lights to my ice bags to keep his beer cold.

YOGA-DOC SAYS . . .

You need to understand a little about inflammation to figure out whether you need to ice or heat an area of pain or injury. Inflammation is a natural, defensive response to tissue damage from an injury, such as an ankle sprain, or an intense physical activity that causes tissue stress but not injury, such as a baseball pitcher throwing one hundred pitches in a game, or anyone who works out hard and feels really stiff the next day or two. Inflammation has five major signs and symptoms: redness, pain, heat, swelling, and loss of function of the injured area. If you have at least one or two of these, then you should *not* use heat. In fact, you should probably use ice 99 percent of the time—unless you have had frostbite in the area of pain.

Ice treatment, or cryotherapy, is the best natural anti-inflammatory on the planet. It helps reduce heat, swelling, and pain without causing damage to your liver, kidneys, or stomach, like most over-the-counter and prescription non-steroidal anti-inflammatories will do. Cryotherapy is also one of the best ways to keep your body from getting stiff and sore after vigorous exercise. Have you ever noticed a baseball pitcher with an ice pack on his shoulder or elbow immediately after a game? This decreases post-exercise recovery time so the athlete can come back and compete as soon as possible with minimal soreness.

Many people ask, "Why shouldn't I use heat on an injured area if it feels so good?" It's true that heat feels good initially, but heat therapy, whether moist or electric, won't pump that inflammation out of your muscles or joints. In fact, heat increases circulation and might cause more inflammatory chemicals to flood the affected area, which results in more stiffness and pain to an injured area and increases the amount of time that it takes to heal. In other words, heat on an injured joint could lock rather than loosen you up. Electric heating pads are known to actually weaken scar tissue or injured muscles by "cooking" or denaturing the proteins in injured muscle, causing decreased stability in the area and increased inflammatory response. Trust me, guys, people with bad backs or necks who refuse to ice but would rather sleep on a heating pad make chiropractic kinesiologists like me crazy. They "undo" all our good work, and then they can't figure out why they're not healing quickly.

So when do you use heat and what type of heat should you use?

Moist heat is great if you have morning stiffness, and no, we're not talking about the "early morning missile crisis." We're talking about arthritic joint pain and stiffness upon waking—without redness, swelling, or loss of function. This type of pain could come from arthritis, like a twenty-year-old injury that has come back for a visit when the barometer drops. If you have these symptoms, then a hot shower will get you going. Back in high school, I developed a ritual of taking a hot shower before each basketball game as a way to warm up my body. It's a ritual I still keep today—except these days, my showers are a lot hotter and a lot longer. The key to preventative maintenance here is to keep your body warm and flexible to decrease the chance of injury.

Today, after a hot shower, I dress in sweats and start right into my YRG workout, which keeps me warm and flexible. If I happen to use some moist heat, I may wrap a warm towel around my back until I'm good and warm from my workout. And trust me, guys, our workout will get you beyond warm in no time at all!

ORGANIC FOODS

Let's put it like this: You take a vegetable that's grown in today's soil, which isn't clean (the way your great-grandfather's soil was before all the pesticides), and then you take that vegetable and spray pesticides on it and then spray enhancers, and then, for extra measure, you spray on some preservatives—and *guess what*? Your veggie may have half the vitamins, minerals, and enzymes than an organic one has. Now cook it, and, well, you might as well eat the napkin in front of you because you will get the same amount of nutrition. Okay, maybe that's a little stiff, but it's close. Most people have no idea what the hell they are eating today, especially all of us raised in this processed food world.

You see, as you've now heard me say many times, I didn't even start my career as a professional wrestler until I was thirty-five years old, so I had to find ways to hold back the hands of time. I found that a healthy diet could help slow those hands down. I also found that the rule "everything in moderation" was even better. The strength of our digestive system is the key to how we assimilate and synthesize our food/fuel and turn it into energy. The better we take care of our digestive system, which consists of the stomach, the small intestines, and the colon, the longer and stronger we live. The key? It's the quality of the fuel that we put into our bodies that gives us the energy to fight the fight and win the war against time. And if you put the purest, most nutrient-rich food into your body to cleanse and heal your digestive system, then all the organs and bodily systems can run more efficiently.

YOGA-DOC SAYS . . .

The food pyramid folks suggest that you eat five to seven or even nine servings of fruit and vegetables per day to receive your Recommended Daily Allowance of nutrients and fiber in your diet. Organically grown fruit and vegetables are pesticide free, hence healthier for you; plus, they give you the highest vitamin, mineral, and natural enzyme content of any food on the planet. They give you the most *bang* for your buck! Now that you know this, why would you want to put anything but organically grown foods in your tank?

Why Organic Juice?

I'm willing to bet that most of the Regular Guys throughout the United States don't get five to nine servings of organic fruits and veggies per day. If they did, they'd have no room for chips, beef, fish, chicken wings, brats, and beer. But sooner or later we have to look at our diet and see which foods are our everyday staples and which ones need to move to the "special occasion" column. Don't get me wrong: I eat a lot of protein (chicken, steak, and fish), but I also balance it with all the fruits and veggies that I can consume. Plus, I drink a lot of *fresh* organic juice to get all that I need from the fruit and veggie group, and more.

What if you could get a whole bunch of vital nutrients—in a less bulky form—with so many vitamins, minerals, and pure energy that you feel like you knocked back a double shot of espresso every time you drank it? Fresh organic juicing will do it for you, and it's so much better for you than the quick high you get from caffeine and all those energy drinks.

YOGA-DOC SAYS . . .

Every time we put caffeine into our bodies, we are burdening our livers and adrenal glands to function at a much higher level of performance than they should. Organic juice gives you a supermarket aisle full of nutrients that feed your body, giving you more energy without pounding the hell out of your liver and adrenals. Organic juice is also a strong detoxifier and blood purifier because of all the antioxidants and natural enzymes it contains. Enzymes from plant sources are now being studied to see how they can be instrumental in curing some of the worst diseases and degenerative disorders that plague us.

I'm going to tell you how I got involved in organic juicing. You see, my grandfather got cancer, and my brother Rory, who was a chiropractor at the time and an organic food enthusiast, decided he was going to go to Mexico to find an alternative to chemotherapy. When my brother came back, he had learned how to make the body an unfriendly place for cancer by utilizing organic juicing. Of course, my grandfather, being the "old school kraut" that he was, had nothing to do with it. Rory tried to explain what he found to me, and I, of course, did the same as my grandfather—I blew him off as well.

So what happened? Why the change? Well, one day I went to a Tony Robbins seminar (Tony has inspired me on many occasions), and at some point, he got on the subject of getting some kind of greens supplement into our systems on a daily basis to energize our bodies. What started to hook me was, of course, how passionate Tony was about this greens supplement, but what sealed the deal was when he said that he didn't care if we bought his product or not. So that day, I bought Tony's greens supplement, and oh my God, did that stuff taste like shit! The next day I went to the health food store to try some other products, and I found one that was pretty good. I used it for a while, and I was definitely feeling a difference in my energy levels.

Then one day, I went down to West Palm Beach for a wrestling show. My dad (Diamond Dallas Dad or DDD, as he likes to be called) lives in the area, and he came over to see me for lunch. When DDD got there, he handed me this jar of purple juice and told me to drink it before we left.

"What is it?" I asked. He said, "Just drink it." I asked, "Why is it purple? Is it grape juice?" He said, "No, there are beets in it." I said, "I hate beets!" He said, "*Just drink it.*" So to shut him up, I did. And you know what? It wasn't that bad. As a matter of fact, I actually liked it.

When I got back to Atlanta, I told my brother about my juice experience with DDD. Rory reminded me that he had told me about organic juicing years ago. "Why would you want to drink all that 'artificial power drink crap' when you can have the best-tasting, high energy, healing organic juice instead?" Now, the one thing that I haven't told you was that over all my years in wrestling, we were constantly tested for everything from AIDS to hepatitis. During my first six years in wrestling, I would constantly have problems with my platelet count. It was so bad that sometimes it actually kept me from wrestling.

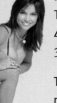

HOT TIP!

The juice recipe Dallas's brother made up for him includes:
40 pounds of carrots, 10 cucumbers, 15 beets, 5 bunches of parsley, 5 bunches of celery, 3 heads of kale, 2 bunches of spinach, 8 red apples, and 4 green apples

This makes about 14 to 17 quarts of juice, and Dallas drinks one or two quarts a day. That means he has to mix a batch every two weeks or so. It will usually keep up to 72 hours with 100 percent vitamins and enzymes if you use the Norwalk juicer (see the Resources section on p. 190). You can also freeze it up to 3 months.

I started juicing about six years ago, and since then, I haven't had a problem with my platelet count or any other type of problem with my blood whatsoever. As a matter of fact, the last time I got my blood work done, my doctor called and asked me what I was doing differently: I had the cleanest blood of anyone he has tested over the age of twenty-five! I was pretty jacked to hear that.

And the only thing I can attribute that to is my juicing. Like all things I do, it is a ritual to me. In other words, I do it whenever possible. The best part is that I have been sick only once in the past six years.

YOGA-DOC SAYS . . .

According to Dr. Norman Walker, a naturopathic doctor, researcher, and pioneer in the field of organic juicing for the restoration and maintenance of health, juicing can be instrumental in dissolving gallstones, arterial plaque, and kidney stones, as well as shrinking and/or preventing certain types of tumors. (See the Resources section on page 190.) Here are just some of the ways the vegetable juice can enhance your health:

Carrot juice is one of the most powerful tools for balancing each system of the body. From the eyes to the liver and gall bladder, from the skin and immune system to the reproductive system, carrot juice can help it all run smoothly. It is very rich in vitamins A, B, C, E, and K, as well as the minerals sodium, potassium, calcium, magnesium, and iron. Carrot juice is the main ingredient in most juicing recipes because it enhances the taste and the positive nutritive effects of almost every other type of fruit or veggie. (Some of the other dark leafy green juices can taste pretty nasty if ingested alone.)

Celery juice is rich in natural organic sodium, magnesium, and iron. It works well with many other vegetable juices and enhances their healing effects.

Cucumber juice is a natural diuretic that also has a cooling and soothing effect on the body's systems and has about 300 enzymes.

Beet juice is a very powerful liver cleanser and a great blood purifier. It tastes great too!

Kale and cabbage juices are incredibly healthy for the digestive system and are also high in vitamin C, sulphur, natural chlorine, and iodine.

Parsley juice is great for the arteries and veins, the kidneys, and the bladder. It is a strong herb—a little bit goes a long way.

Spinach juice is incredible for the entire digestive system and most other bodily systems. It is very high in vitamins C and E, as well as a good source of iron. (Remember how spinach gave Popeye the energy to kick Bluto's ass each time they threw down?)

Organic apple juice is high in all vitamins and minerals, as well as water content. It tastes great and speeds up the absorption of almost any vegetable juice that it is mixed with.

Juice Machines—What's the Difference?

The juicer most people know is "The Juice Man Juicer." Do you remember the guy who's about eighty years old, with wild eyebrows and way too much energy? Well, his juicer is fine if you want to juice every single time you want some juice. The reality is, that's a pain in the ass. To be honest, juicing in general is a real pain in the ass, but the benefits outweigh the pain when it comes to preventative maintenance.

Most juicers out there are all the same. They cost a few hundred dollars, they grind up the vegetables, and spit out the juice. The problem is that after twenty minutes, the juice starts to lose vitamins and enzymes, so you have to drink the juice right away, and you can't freeze it.

The juicer I have cuts up the veggies into little pieces and then squeezes the juice out of those veggies so that there are no vitamins or enzymes left over. It all goes into your glass. What I love about my juicer is that because of its extraction process, you get about one-third more juice, which lasts for up to 72 hours in your refrigerator, with 100 percent of the vitamins, minerals, and enzymes. You can also freeze the rest of what you have juiced for up to 3 months. You can't do this with any other juicers.

Organic Juicing and YRG

Now check this out: The Yoga for Regular Guys Workout is the "Organic Juicing of Exercise Programs." Why? Because we already know that YRG is the most time-efficient stretching, strengthening, and heart-healthy stress-release exercise program all wrapped up into one. The deep breathing and deep stretching postures push more oxygen (the element most essential for life) into every crease, crevice, corner, and cell of your body. This allows for more efficient blood purification, organ cleansing, and overall brain and body coordination.

YOGA-DOC SAYS . . .
When you inhale deeply while stretching and twisting into each yoga position, you are pushing oxygen-rich blood into each organ while opening blocked areas of the body that may have been compromised from years of bad posture, previous traumas, and scar tissue build-up related to those traumas. Oxygen- and nutrient-rich blood also speeds up the internal detoxification process and allows the energy that your body has produced from your organic juicing to be utilized more efficiently and effectively. So your Yoga for Regular Guys workout is organic juicing's ultimate Tag Team Partner!

CHIROPRACTIC AND APPLIED KINESIOLOGY

The body is like a car, and when it isn't running as smoothly as it should, it needs a tune-up from outside help. This is where chiropractors and applied kinesiologists come in. They can help you supplement the good work you are doing on your own with your YRG work-outs. These guys help keep you on top of your game. They are not only important when you take some rough bumps in life, they should also be key players in your new preventative maintenance program.

DDP's Humpty Dumpty Days

Back in the glory days of World Championship Wrestling (now under the WWE banner), when I came off the road after a week or more of bouncing my body around the world, I would gather all the king's horses and all the king's men to put DDP back together again. Every time I came off the road, I would first go to the gym and get my workout in. Then I would go right to my chiropractor/applied kinesiologist, Dr. Ken West. This guy is a master; he's the Yoda of kinesiologists. I would typically spend up to two hours on his table. Then I would head right over to one of my massage therapists. Those were what I call my "Humpty Dumpty Days," and they were the only way this old boy kept going.

Putting Humpty Dumpty Back Together

Dr. West led the group of healthcare specialists that helped put Humpty Dumpty back together again after each show—and fast, so I could get back into the ring after taking some nasty bumps.

The best example of Dr. West's expertise came in May 2000 when I was wrestling Jeff Jarrett for the world championship title, in *not one*, *not two*, but *THREE* steel cages, stacked one on top of the other. If you saw my movie classic *Ready to Rumble*, you know the cage I'm talking about. Except in this case, there were no running cameras or a director yelling "Cut!" This match was *live*, in front of twenty thousand screaming fans.

Jeff and I had gone to the arena the night before our match to look at this monster of a cage and go over the stunts we were going to do. The cage was forty-five feet high and divided into cages on three separate levels. To get from the first cage to the second we had to use a twelve-foot ladder. The outer cage was fenced in with cables running through the fencing so that we could walk, run, or fall on top of it. The cages were built with steel pip-ing around the perimeter for strength. In one of the corners, there was a one-foot by two-foot rectangular shaped hole, which was there to get us from the first cage to the second. (By the way, no wrestling company does crazy shit like this anymore.)

The scene was the Kemper Arena in Kansas City. We were about to do a high-risk match with aerial stunts in the very same arena where, almost one year to the day, Owen Hart had fallen to his death while sailing in toward the ring on a high wire. Owen was one of the nicest guys I had ever met in the wrestling business, and I have to tell you, I was a little spooked by the whole deal.

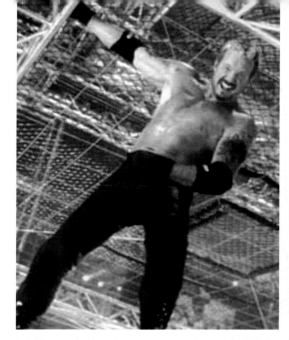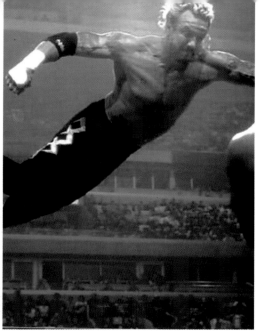

Left: The three-level steel cage from Kemper Arena; right: DDP flies off the top rope with twenty thousand people in the background.

The first hour Jeff and I were up in the three-story cage, going over our upcoming match, I was very tentative. By the second hour, I felt a little better. By the third hour, I was feeling so familiar with the structure that I felt like I could do cartwheels in the damn thing. As you could guess, being that comfortable on something that dangerous is not always a good thing. I remember telling Jeff about a stunt that I wanted to do where we were on the second floor of the cage and I was going to run him into one of the cage walls. That wall would fall down (which would really shock the hell out of the fans because it would appear that we were going to fall thirty feet to the ground), but in actuality, we would only knock the wall on the top of the first cage ceiling. Then, we would fight around the second cage level until we started up for the third, which is where the world championship title belt was located.

At the time I was describing this to Jeff, he was standing on the third level looking down at me. I was on the second level, looking up and laying out the stunt. You have to understand, we had never done a match like this before—no one had! So you can understand that Jeff was a little apprehensive. Jeff asked, "What do we do after the wall drops down? Where do we think we should go from there?"

I looked up and answered, "Well Bro, we just—" and I turned to show him what would be a good next move. As I turned around, I fell through the rectangular hole in the floor of the second cage. My right leg dropped a hundred miles an hour through that hole and I caught my right shoulder on the opposite side of the hole. Jeff looked down in disbelief and asked if I was all right, and I honestly didn't know. I felt a jolt go through my body like I had never felt before. I was hanging in this hole, motionless, and for a few moments, I thought I might have

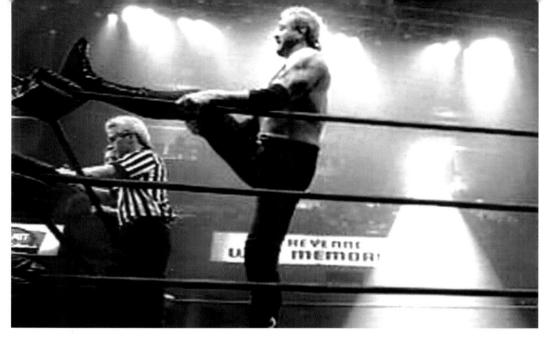

Back in 1999 while filming *Ready to Rumble*, DDP had to stick his leg on the top rope to get any kind of stretch.

broken my neck. As Jeff asked me again if I was all right, I started to move my fingers and toes, and realized that I was all right—but not really. So I began to lower myself down to the floor.

The boys took me back to the hotel and put me in bed, where I immediately started to ice my body. I took a couple of painkillers and passed out around 11 PM. At 5 AM I woke up, but I literally couldn't move. I had to go to the bathroom, but I couldn't move. So I fell on the ground and crawled on my stomach to the bathroom. When I pulled myself back in bed, I called Janie Engel, the Radar O'Reilly of WCW, and told her that I needed Dr. Ken West to come out and fix me, or there would be *no main event* for this PPV.

Through the grace of God, somehow I got a hold of Doc West in Atlanta and he flew straight out to save me. A couple of the boys literally carried me to my car and then into the Kemper Arena. The doc got there at 2:30 PM and worked on me for more than five hours. I'm telling you, I couldn't walk at 2:30 PM, but if you ever get a chance to see that match, you would never know just how hurt I was. The doc worked on me after the match and then again the next morning. He got me to the point where I was also able to make it to Nitro that Monday night.

A Closer Look at Chiropractors and Kinesiologists

Now, I've been treated by chiropractors of all different types for many years, and some of my closest friends are chiropractors. Hell, even my brother, Rory, is a doctor of chiropractic. But please understand that not all "bone docs" are the same. So my best advice to everyone is to make friends with a chiropractor who is a sports extremity specialist, or even better, an applied kinesiologist, like Doc West and the Yoga-Doc. These guys have gone above and beyond their traditional chiropractic education to become the true body mechanics that we need to keep us tuned up, rotated, and balanced for the next big race. The Yoga-Doc will tell you a little about what makes each one different, but the bottom line is, these guys help keep you on top of your game. They are not only important when you take some rough bumps in life, they should also be key players in your new preventative maintenance program.

YOGA-DOC SAYS . . .

Chiropractic is one of the most cost-effective treatments for back pain, neck pain, headaches, whiplash injuries, and carpal tunnel syndrome, but it is also a well-known fact that chiropractic care is one of the best ways to assure that your musculo-skeletal system is working at its optimal level of performance. Chiropractors adjust misaligned joints in the spine and extremities to restore lost function, decrease muscle spasms, and re-establish proper blood flow and nerve flow to each area of the body. The positive effects of chiropractic adjustments are decreased pain and the ability to use your body to its maximum capability, without structural impediment.

As DDP stated, all chiropractors are not created equal, so here's the inside info on what to look for in a good doctor of chiropractic:

First and foremost, you will want to steer clear of any chiropractor wearing a white lab coat—a dead giveaway that the chiropractor is insecure about what he does and that he is trying to fool you into believing that he is some type of medical doctor.

You will also want to bypass the chiropractor who claims that he or she can help almost any problem by adjusting only one or two of the uppermost vertebrae in your neck. They call themselves "upper cervical specialists" and utilize the Atlas Orthogonal, Grostic, Blair, NUCCA, or upper cervical specific techniques. These "Atlas only" chiropractors are working with a very small toolbox, so they are okay for your run-of-the-mill headache or neck pain, but they are very limited when it comes to offering structural rehabilitation exercises, healthy lifestyle advice, or caring for sports- or work-related injuries.

You guys want the one-stop shop for all your structural needs. Look for doctors who have one of three designations or advanced chiropractic certifications, such as the Sports Extremity Practitioners, known as Certified Chiropractic Extremity Practitioners (CCEPs), Certified Chiropractic Sports Practitioners (CCSPs), and/or Applied Kinesiologists.

Applied Kinesiology, or AK, is an extensive discipline of examining and treating functional health problems through manual muscle testing, traditional chiropractic adjustments, muscle release and strengthening techniques, traditional craniopathy, and principles of acupuncture. AK also offers dietary advice along with personalized recommendations for herbal and vitamin supplementation to best serve each patient in a holistic manner.

Hey, guys, if all the top sports programs in the country use AK and sports chiropractors to keep them at their best, then why shouldn't you? Like I said, what the hell, GIVE IT A SHOT!

Massage Therapy

Massage therapy is extremely important for your preventative maintenance program and goes hand in hand with chiropractic care and your YRG workouts. As you already know, I use massage as an integral part of my "Humpty Dumpty Days" when I have to get put back together after a tough match. But I also recommend at least one massage per month for general stress relief.

It may take you a while to find a great massage therapist, but once you find one, you'll never want him or her to move away. Finding the right therapist depends on what you like and need. Some guys will only work with a female, but she will have to be strong enough to work out all your knots and trigger points. So you might be looking for a therapist who is one part angel and one part sadist. Other guys don't mind what gender their therapist is as long as they get a great massage.

YOGA-DOC SAYS . . .

Massage therapy has different benefits, including stress relief, increased blood and lymph circulation, more efficient toxin removal from sore and stiff muscles, as well as pain relief and better mobility. Massage therapy, like chiropractic care, helps balance all of the body's systems, thereby increasing immune system function and allowing for better homeostasis.

There are many massage techniques, including Swedish and sports massage, which are more relaxing, as well as more vigorous and deep-tissue techniques, such as NeuroMuscular Therapy and Rolfing. There are more meditative and esoteric techniques, such as Polarity therapy, Cranio-Sacral therapy, and Reiki therapy. There are also assisted stretching techniques, such as Zen Shiatsu and Thai massage therapy. My recommendation would be to find a versatile massage therapist who is well versed in the relaxing, deep tissue, and stretching styles of massage and allow them to show you the ropes. The good news is that almost any type of massage is better than nothing, so enjoy the journey!

EATING FOR HEALTHY WEIGHT LOSS

First of all, let's get one thing straight. The proper way to lose weight is not to go on a diet. How many people have you seen go on a diet, lose a ton of weight, and then a year later, they are fatter than they were before they started the diet? Why didn't they keep the weight off? Well, for starters, they used the word *diet*, and diets don't work, because once you stop dieting, the tendency is to bounce right back to beer keg belly territory in no time. The bottom line is that if you really want to lose weight, get in shape, and keep in shape, you have to lose the diet and decide to change your *lifestyle* instead.

When someone uses the word *diet*, they are describing a temporary eating program (which may or may not be healthy) that will be used to reach a certain weight goal, which, once attained, will be discarded for the old habits that made them a fat cow in the first place. A diet might help you lose some weight, but it's the lifestyle modifications that you continually adhere to that help you keep off what you lose. Healthy eating is the perfect complement to your YRG workouts; if you decide to stick to both, the positive effects can be permanent.

The battle of the big belly is fought using the weapons of dietary changes, exercise, and most importantly, discipline. Your diet turns into a healthy lifestyle once the application of discipline becomes an ingrained habit. This book has given you the exercise program. In the next chapter, we will also inspire you to stay focused and disciplined, but now, we'll talk a little about the healthy eating part of your lifestyle that can take you the rest of the way.

YOGA-DOC SAYS . . .

Almost everybody has heard something about the Atkins Diet, a high-protein, very low-carb and moderate- to high-fat program. This diet relies very heavily on the process of *ketosis*, which is when the body uses what it needs from the intake of protein and then converts any excess protein into the minimum amount of carbohydrate necessary to run the body. The less the amount of carbohydrates consumed, the less fatty deposits that will be stored in the body. So, you might be asking, what falls into the carbohydrate category, anyway? Cookies, ice cream, candy, cakes, potatoes, chips, any type of bread, rice, pasta, beer, wine, liquor (sorry), soda, juice, fruit, veggies, and absolutely everything with sugar. Many people have lost weight on this diet. But it is definitely a short-term eating program and certainly not a lifestyle program that can be sustained, because this diet can be quite stressful on the kidneys and may also cause an increase in blood cholesterol and triglyceride levels.

I've had many patients who have been very successful using a more moderate low-carb diet known as the South Beach Diet. This eating program can be used on a more long-term basis, but it is not for anyone who has dairy sensitivities. The Zone Diet is a time-tested and very successful lifestyle program that can be sustained for an indefinite period for those who stick with it. It is based on eating meals that are 40 percent carbohydrate, 30 percent protein, and 30 percent fat.

I've had patients who have reported sustainable weight loss by simply cutting their portions down by 25 to 30 percent per meal without changing anything else. I like to eat four or five small meals per day that consist of mostly protein and vegetables. I recommend that you eat your biggest meal of the day at breakfast or lunch, because your body is more likely to store what you eat for dinner as fat. This is because we have a tendency to be less active at night, so our bodies won't have as much of a need for instant energy. I have a favorite saying, "If you want to gain weight, just eat late." Now, listen guys, it's hard to eat right all the time, but I find that if I eat right for eight out of every ten meals, I'm a happy guy.

The Yoga-Doc pretty much hit things right on the head when it comes to eating to lose weight and stay in shape. And now, I'm going to even make it easier for you.

If you're trying to lose that tire around your stomach or lose weight in general, immediately start writing down everything you eat and drink and what *time* you ate and drank it. Writing down what you eat and drink makes you accountable for your actions. I will really get into this subject in the next chapter. When you write down what you are eating and what time you are eating it, you will definitely see what you are dealing with when it comes to the changes you need to make.

You should always eat your carbohydrates before your proteins because your stomach and small intestines will always attempt to break down and absorb the carbs first. Carbohydrates are digested the quickest to supply the body with instant energy as well as enough fuel to help you digest whatever else you eat. Yes, it takes energy to digest all that food that we pile into our bodies. This is why many folks get very tired after a meal.

So if you happen to eat your proteins and good fats before your carbs, your digestive system will give the carbohydrates priority, which will cause the proteins and fats to sit in your stomach until all those carbs are broken down and absorbed. This is not the healthiest scenario for your digestive tract.

The most important meal of the day for me is breakfast. Every morning I make ten eggs to make sure I get my protein. That's right, ten eggs. Now, five of those yolks I throw away because I don't want all the extra cholesterol, but I do want the protein. Even though I eat these eggs every day, I never eat those eggs exactly the same way. One day, I may have them with cheddar cheese and ketchup, the next, it could be with corn, mushrooms, onions, artichokes, salsa, black beans, cream cheese, or you name it. There are so many ways to eat eggs in a healthy way and make them taste great that some day, I'm going to put out a cookbook called *Cooking for Regular Guys*. In addition to my eggs, I also have two pieces of Ezekiel 4:9 Cinnamon Raisin bread. Ezekiel 4:9 is not your regular type of bread. It looks like regular bread, but it is actually 100 percent flourless, sprouted whole-grain bread. It's a complete protein, and it's absolutely delicious.

Sometimes, I may even have a bowl of certified organic multigrain hot cereal; if you add blueberries, cranberries, cut apples, peaches, pine nuts, walnuts, or anything else you like to the cereal, it will taste incredible. My bros come over all the time for breakfast because they know they are never going to get the same thing twice.

YOGA-DOC SAYS . . .
You may not get the healthy and organic ingredients if you are eating on the road, but you can try to duplicate DDP's "Mega Breakfast" even when traveling. You should see the terrified looks on the faces of our waitresses when we order breakfast at the Cracker Barrel restaurant.

The rest of the day I try to eat as much chicken, steak (cow or buffalo), and fish as possible. If I'm going to eat carbs, I do it in the morning or afternoon, because I still have time to burn them off. I try to combine all of these meals with some kind of vegetable or salad, but sometimes because I take in so many veggies with my juicing, I'll just eat my protein by itself, though never without some kind of seasoning or marinade on it.

You see, guys, I eat pretty damn healthy. But if it didn't taste good or great, there is no way that I would continue to eat healthy. I believe it has to taste good if I am ever going to stay in this type of ritual, which has become my *lifestyle*.

LAST BUT NOT LEAST: WATER

Did you ever wake up with a nasty hangover and dry mouth that felt like someone emptied dirty cat litter in your face while you were sleeping? Or did you ever have your heat turned up nice and high on a cold night and woke up dried out and feelin' shitty? Well guys, dehydration is the culprit, and the answer is simple: Drink more water—your health depends upon it!

There is air, and then there is water. They are both essential to life. Air is everywhere, and sometimes, it's even clean enough to breathe. The problem is, most of us don't drink enough water each day. But why is water so important and how much do we really need?

YOGA-DOC SAYS . . .

Our bodies are composed of roughly 60 to 70 percent water, and if we begin to dehydrate even slightly, our muscles will become weaker and less responsive, our blood volume will decrease (not a good thing), and every function from nutrient transport to waste removal and from acid/base balance to hormone regulation could be impaired. Unfortunately, our thirst signal doesn't set off the alarm until we are 1 to 2 percent dehydrated. This is too late if we plan on being our best at all times. We need to drink at least 3 to 4 quarts of clean water throughout the day but preferably between meals, whether we feel thirsty or not.

I mention clean water because, no matter where you may be reading this book, you can bet that the tap water in your location is neither clean nor pure. The saying used to be, if you go to Mexico, don't drink the water. I like to say, don't drink the tap water anywhere unless you want a bacteria, treated sewage, and chlorine cocktail! Your best bet is to find some kind of water purification system. Carbon filtration or reverse osmosis systems are time tested and do a more than adequate job. Bottled water that's labeled filtered, purified, ozonated, or distilled is also very good.

Another way to make sure that you are properly hydrated is to check to see if your urine is clear rather than yellow. If your urine is clear and you are visiting the restroom a minimum of six times per day, then *you're* in the clear.

Water acts like coolant for your car. It helps regulate your body temperature whether you're sitting on the couch or doing Yoga for Regular Guys. And if you happen to be sweating your ass off doing the YRG workout, then you need to replace those lost fluids—and no, coffee, soda, and beer don't count. In fact, any drink with sugar, caffeine, or alcohol actually dehydrates you. Now you know what causes that morning hangover!

I like to drink at least a gallon or two of filtered or purified water per day. I have a water filter at home, but when I'm on the road, I always buy enough bottled water to keep me well hydrated. And trust me guys, air travel dries you out more than you can imagine, so drink as much bottled water as possible before, during, and after you fly.

There is an added bonus to all this water business. When you drink plenty of water, you are also helping your body flush toxins and emulsify fat out of your system. So guys, your best bet is to keep it wet!

I have been lucky enough to find a lot of services and products to help me change my lifestyle for the better. For the goods on this information, turn to the Resources section on p. 190.

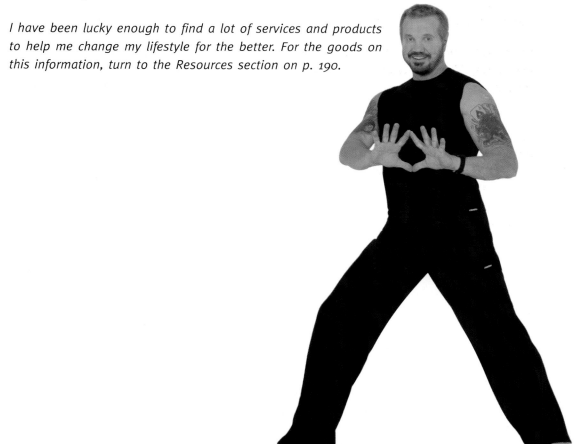

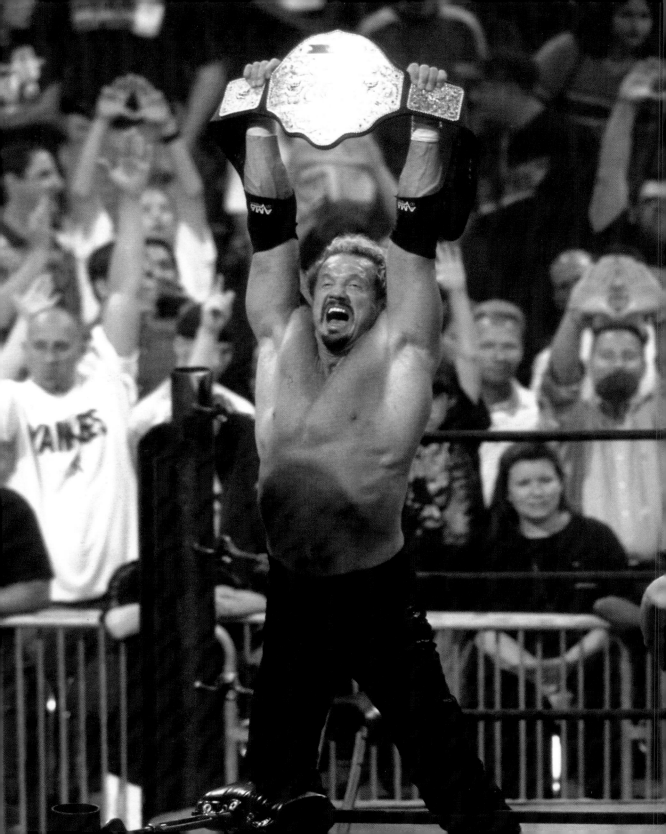

CHAPTER 5

INSPIRATION, MOTIVATION, AND CONGRATULATIONS

I have been calling myself the master of *motivation*, *inspiration*, and *stimulation* since the first time I stepped into the square circle back in 1988 as a wrestling manager. You see, back then I thought I was too old to start to wrestle. I was thirty-one at the time—what the hell was I thinking?

Of those three words, I believe *inspiration* is the best. Why? Because inspiration comes from within each and every one of us. It comes from the inside out. I can motivate you all I want, but when I'm gone, the passionate and motivational words I used to fire you up will stay with you only as long as you can keep them in the forefront of your mind. When you are truly inspired, you can do anything.

Take a look at Ted Evans, my favorite Regular Guy who does YRG. This guy truly inspires me. He's a real man's man! Ted first started doing yoga at the age of sixty-six. Earlier in his youth he crushed one of his vertebrae and damaged three of his discs. He kept active in the face of all his physical challenges and then, at the young age of sixty-six, made a decision to start doing yoga. Now to me, that's pretty damn inspirational!

 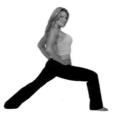

◄ This is the first time DDP was awarded the World Championship title, in Tacoma, Washington, in 1999.

A YRG STORY OF INSPIRATION

I was the first Regular Guy Ted ever saw do yoga, and I was no kid at the time; I was forty-three. We both worked out at the same gym, and over the period of a year, he watched my flexibility and strength increase month in and month out. One day he came up and asked me a few questions about exactly what I was doing. I explained the basics, and pretty much forgot about the incident.

Flash forward to about three years later, when I called the Yoga-Doc and asked him if he wanted to be involved in the project I was calling "Yoga for Regular Guys." The Yoga-Doc was all for it, even after I explained that his involvement in YRG might just make him the black sheep of the "serious" yoga crowd. That only made him laugh out loud. He said, "Hey, Dallas—as far as the hairy granola yoga folk are concerned, they already don't like me because I'm the *yoga for jocks* guy. And as long as we get a few hundred thousand Regular Guys doing yoga, I'm in!"

We worked tirelessly on developing both the YRG program and helping me develop as a YRG teacher. The funniest thing about all of this was the first time I ever taught the YRG work-out in a group setting, I tag-teamed it with the Yoga-Doc during one of his weekly yoga classes. It was about a year ago, and I didn't take much notice of anybody in the class because I was so preoccupied with how I was going to teach this thing. I had never taught a full class before. But the chemistry the Yoga-Doc and I had was unbelievable. It was like we had been doing it for years.

Once we got into the flow of it, I looked to the back of the class and noticed Ted. I stopped right in the middle of the class while we were in a standing position and said, "Hey, Bro. Wow, you've really come a long way!" I found out that Ted had picked up with the Yoga-Doc's class shortly after we had that conversation about yoga three years earlier.

When we planned our photo shoot for this book, I asked the Yoga-Doc to make sure that we got Ted a plane ticket. I definitely wanted this guy in the book. But the Yoga-Doc told me Ted had just undergone surgery on his knee two weeks earlier. I said, "Well, we're not shooting for another two weeks. Do you think he could be ready?" Yoga-Doc said, "Dude, this guy is seventy years old. I wouldn't bet on it." And then we both laughed our asses off.

But when it came time for the photo shoot, I'll be damned if the tough SOB wasn't ready. Four weeks after his surgery, I flew Ted out to LA from Atlanta to be a part of the YRG workout. And to no one's surprise, he did it like the warrior that he is. Now *that's* inspirational! No one can ever tell me that they're too old or too beat up to do YRG.

MAKING A DECISION

I want to give you guys a goal. You see, if you don't know where you're going, how the hell are you ever going to get there?

But we need to be clear about something first. Before you can even set a goal, you have to make a decision. Making a decision is the most important thing you can do. Why? Because the true meaning of the word *decide* can get you to the Promised Land. You see, most people don't really make true decisions. The Latin root of *decide* means "to cut off all possibility." So a person who actually made a true decision to accomplish something would have no alternative but to do what they decided.

It all comes down to the difference between "hoping" something is going to happen and "knowing" something is going to happen. Think about your goal and just "hope" that it's going to happen. When you just hope for something to happen, the picture isn't clear, the colors aren't that bright, and the vision isn't that exact.

Contrast that with what happens when you "know" a future goal is going to occur. You expect it, and you know with absolute certainty that it will come. The picture is very clear, the colors are very bright and vivid, and the vision is very exact, specific, and focused. Try this with something you want. How about getting into the best shape you have ever been, using the YRG workout? Visualize yourself doing the 20-Minute Workout three times a week. Remember, *everyone has twenty minutes!*

After you have made a *decision*, you have to put it to work . . .

Applying Your Decision

The formula we are going to be using is called SMACK:

S: SPECIFY
M: MONITOR
A: ACHIEVE
C: CHOOSE
K: KEEP IT GOING

Specify: Know exactly what you want to accomplish with your YRG workout. Let's say for example that you want to lose thirty-six pounds—wow!!! That's a shit-load of weight to lose. But if you know that you are going to change your lifestyle by sticking with your workout and dropping the weight, then the weight will come off! This can work with any goal, from building more muscle mass to gaining greater flexibility—just be specific about your goal.

Monitor: Monitor your progress by breaking your goal down into doable increments. Break a year down into months. So if your goal is to lose thirty-six pounds in a year, then you're losing only three pounds a month. That's less than a pound per week! If you are sticking to your YRG workouts, this should not be a problem.

Achieve: To understand whether your goals are truly attainable or not really depends on your lifestyle. Most times, you have to change your lifestyle to achieve your goals. It may be your time management skills that need attention—then again it may just come down to true dedication. Either way, it will come down to what you really want, because once you find that out, you can trust that your goal is attainable. If you are breaking your goal into measurable goals and not setting the bar too high, too fast, you are allowing yourself to really believe you can achieve—and then, well, achievement is possible.

Choose: Are you choosing actions that are compatible with your goal? Now this is a big one. If you're drinking half a case of beer a night, eating crap every night, and slouching on the couch whenever you can, then the answer is absolutely not! But if you're going to live life in moderation, and you have decided to live a healthier lifestyle in combination with your YRG workout sessions, then your actions are definitely compatible with attaining your goal.

Keep it going: This is your ritual. You must discipline yourself to do the work necessary and to do it continuously. Do it each day, without fail. If your goal is to do your YRG twenty minutes per day or twenty minutes three times per week—and trust me, you can do it—then it MUST be done. If you made a real decision and saw the goal in your mind, then you already know that anything is possible!

Last but not least, remember to write down all of your goals. I can't express to you how important this is. Take again, for example, that your goal is to lose weight by practicing your YRG, and of course you have to eat right, too. Write down how much weight you want to lose and in what period of time because this makes you accountable to *you*. Take pictures of yourself from all sides, and measure your body everywhere. (Well, okay guys, maybe not everywhere, but you get the picture.) You want to keep a visual record because, as time goes on, at some point you are going to stop losing weight. Your weight is going to turn to muscle, and you're going to get a little heavier. But that's not a bad thing; it's a good thing, because muscle is more dense and weighs more than fat. The bottom line is that you're going to lose inches, and you'll look and feel better. You'll watch yourself lose weight, get in shape, get flexible, and stay hard.

If you make some real changes, send your testimony to www.diamonddallaspage.com, and we will post your story. You can e-mail me your YRG questions by clicking onto the "Regular Guys Yoga Gurus" section. We will have a running list of the most frequently asked questions on the site, and if yours is a new one that we haven't already answered and it is even semi-intelligent, we'll post it.

REGULAR GUYS WHO AIN'T SO REGULAR

The number one Regular Guy who I would think would never be caught dead doing yoga (besides myself, of course) wrote the foreword to this book. And believe it or not Rob Zombie is a "Regular Guy" who just happens to be a self-made superstar. I know most people would never in a million years think of a guy like Robbie Z doing YRG—and that's the whole point of this book. It's funny, because after a few months of doing YRG with me, people started to notice a difference in Robbie Z's body. People would say, "Damn, Rob, you look great—what are you doing?" He is quite the prankster, and he would milk his answer for all its worth. He would take his time and say, "Well, I'm doing yoga," just waiting for their reply.

"Yoga???" they would ask. "Yeah, yoga." His buddies' replies would almost always be the same: "Isn't that sweeeeet..." RZ would pause a moment or two, and then he'd say, "Yeah—yoga. I'm doing yoga with DIAMOND DALLAS PAGE!" And that would always get the same amazed response: "You mean the *wrestler* Diamond Dallas Page teaches you yoga?"

Absof**kinglutely. I did teach Robbie Z YRG.

I've gotten superstars who also happen to be Regular Guys from all over the world into YRG. Two more of my favorites are the boys from the band Trick Pony. They are the first good old boys I got doing YRG—Ira Dean and Keith Burns. What's great about the boys from Trick Pony is that they came supplied with Heidi, their own yoga-babe, and she is hot. I first met the boys and Heidi back at the best golf charity on the planet, the Price Oil Celebrity Golf Tournament. They were unknown at the time, but today, they are one of country's hottest groups. Ira and Keith were some of the first Regular Guys to get into YRG—it's what keeps them mean and lean.

The Georgia Tech men's basketball team has been doing Yoga for Regular Guys with the Yoga-Doc since the 2001–2002 season. When these guys began, they were cramping up and falling out of their yoga positions. Then DDP and the Yoga-Doc teamed up to give the Yellow Jackets one slobber knocker of a workout! Now they are strong, flexible, balanced, and focused. No wonder they're so successful!

New York Mets Pitcher Kris Benson began doing Yoga for Regular Guys with the Yoga-Doc shortly after the 2004 baseball season. He took to it right away, and is now able to do some seriously strong yoga positions. By the time Kris reported to spring training, he was lean, mean, and ready for a great season ahead!

CONGRATULATIONS

Congratulations! You have finished learning what you need to start a healthier and more ful-filling lifestyle. Now put down this book, get your ass up, and *get to work*. Of course, you're going to have to pick this book back up from time to time to remind yourself about what the hell you're doing, but that's all a part of the process. Have a great time, and enjoy those yoga-babes. Most of all, BE UNSTOPPABLE!

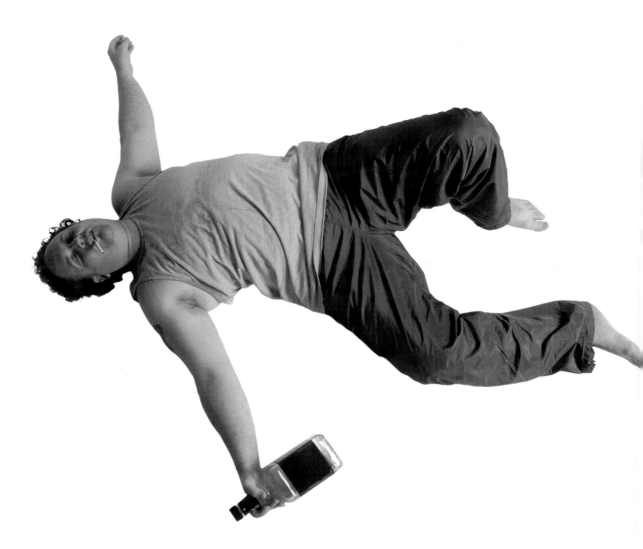

THANKS

I want to thank my wife, Kimberly, for taking an idea I had and making that idea better by making me see it clearly. She's not only hot as hell, she's also a woman of wisdom.

I want to thank Maximo Morrone for jumping on board this project on spec—a.k.a. *no money up front*. You took some AMAZING shots, Max.

I want to thank my manager, Barry Levine, for helping us light the cover shots, loaning your office to us, and offering your creative mind and years of experience while shooting the cover of this book. Also, thank you for having the insight to put me together with Laurie Dolphin. Barry, you're the best!

I want to thank Aaron Blitzstein for his great comical quips in my intro—you are one funny SOB! And of course Rich Schmick and Brian Bentley.

I want to thank Rick Perfetto for supplying most of the real cool workout gear that was worn by the Yoga-Doc, me, and the *gorgeous* yoga-babes.

I want to thank Laurie Dolphin and Allison Meierding at AuthorScape, Inc. I can honestly say that without you two, there would be no book. You ladies are *also* the best! Hugs and kisses to you both! And I don't want to forget Brian Ponto, who silhouetted every photo in this book (good Gawd!).

I want to thank Laurie's man, Stuart, for telling me, with a good buzz mind you, not to peel the vegetables but to wash them. And he was right! We got a third more juice!

And of course, I must thank the Yoga-Doc and his yoga-babe, Jennifer. Yoga-Doc was the best. Of course there were times when he was overworked, irritable, and down-right nasty, and that's why I'm thanking you, Jen—for keeping him sane throughout this project. Great job Yoga-Doc! I could never have done it without you. You're a true bro.

ABOUT THE YRG CREW

Dr. Craig S. Aaron, the "Yoga-Doc," is a sports chiropractor and applied kinesiologist who is also a Certified Chiropractic Extremity Practitioner. Dr. Aaron has been studying and teaching different forms of yoga since 1988, and he is the yoga and flexibility consultant for the Georgia Tech Athletic Department. Dr. Aaron has also worked with many members of the NFL, NBA, Major League Baseball, International Federation of Bodybuilders, and the Senior PGA Tour. He has also trained professional tennis players, and, of course, professional wrestlers. Dr. Aaron is the developer and producer of the video *Dr. Craig Aaron's Extreme Yoga for the Warrior Athlete*, a fun and action-packed program that focuses on functional training for peak athletic performance.

Jennifer Aaron, an aesthetician who specializes in holistic facial skin care, is a fitness enthusiast and yoga instructor. Jennifer started practicing yoga soon after she was introduced to Ashtanga vinyasa by her husband, Dr. Craig Aaron. She loved the sense of renewed mental and physical vigor she got from her classes. Jennifer is entering her seventh year of practice in this ancient healing art form. She was certified by one of the country's most renowned yoga teachers, David Swenson.

Christi Bauerlee is a country singer (her album can be heard on www.christibauerlee.com). Christi almost lost her little brother, Ted, to a traumatic brain injury caused by a car accident, a tragedy that would become a turning point in her life. She gave up everything to be by his side with her family. She believes that prayer, love, faith, and music contributed to her brother's survival, and that encouraging Ted to become involved with yoga will help him regain his health both physically and mentally.

André Brooks reached elite international levels in amateur boxing. With four Golden Gloves championships under his belt, his wise mother insisted: "Hang up the gloves, and save all your marbles while you still have them." André took her advice and completed an intensive training program, graduating from Precision Beauty School to become the original "Boxing Beautician." Today, along with his active work and study of theater, film, and television, he continues teaching fitness and boxing classes in Hollywood during the evenings. André also stays busy in his spare time with his work as a hairstylist. The "Boxing Beautician"—one of a kind!

Dorothy Dawn, R.D., is a dietitian and author of the book *The Best Darn Book About Health and Nutrition*. Her book stresses the importance of balancing the physical, mental, and spiritual aspects of health. Dorothy has lectured at Santa Ana College in Southern California and is also a consultant and speaker for various organizations and corporations.

Tye Dorsey's passion for dance, jiu jitsu, and capoeira led her to study throughout Germany, South Korea, Brazil, and many other exotic locales. While teaching English in Japan, Tye encountered yoga. She enjoys its emphasis on flexibility and strength, and is enthusiastic about sharing this learning with others. She lives, in sunny L.A., by the maxim: "What would you do if you knew you couldn't fail?"

Ted Evans has been active all his life. Even a fracture of one of the vertebrae in his upper thoracic spine didn't slow him down for long. Ted has always been quite strong, but he noticed that his flexibility was decreasing as he aged. In 2000, Ted saw DDP doing some yoga stretches at a gym in Atlanta and decided that he too needed to give yoga a shot to increase his flexibility and overall health. At age sixty-six, Ted began to take yoga classes with the Yoga-Doc. Since then, he has made many gains in flexibility, strength, and balance, while he continues to stand out as a true inspiration to his teachers and fellow students.

Bruce Fennigkoh entered the U.S. Navy after high school, learned to weld—and traveled the world. After nine years, he left the Navy with a skill, an associates' degree, a desire to learn, and a new wife. He studied at San Diego State University Army Reserve Officers Training Corps in 1987 and completed his bachelor's degree and Army Officer Basic Course. After eleven years of civilian life, Bruce returned to active duty in the active guard reserve program and now works at several units in the Los Angeles area. He finds yoga is the solution to keeping fit and relieving the tensions that come in his busy life.

Gypsy is a professional dancer in Los Angeles, California. She has studied many dance forms, as well as gymnastics, yoga, and pilates. She is now teaching a class called "Take It Off" and continues performing with her dance troupe, The Green Eyed Ladies.

Kimberly Page has always maintained an avid interest in health and fitness. For several years, Kimberly joined her husband in the professional wrestling industry, playing the role of his on-screen wife and manager. Later she developed the Nitro Girls, a popular dance team for the show. Currently, she is an actress and model and has appeared in films such as *Seabiscuit* and *Rat Race*; her television appearances include *Live with Regis and Kathie Lee*, *Entertainment Tonight*, *Extra*, and *Hollywood Squares*. She has also appeared in national publications, including *Playboy*, *Maxim*, *Stuff*, *Muscle & Fitness*, *Ironman*, and *TV Guide*.

Alan Rackley found yoga at a crucial time in his life. He weighed three hundred pounds and was experiencing the many negative effects of obesity: back pain, knee pain, bouts of high blood pressure, blood sugar problems, and sleep apnea. Wisely, he bought a DVD of a yoga routine and started to practice yoga. Over a few months, this led to some initial weight loss, and he started to feel better about himself. Yoga, combined with better eating habits, led to an amazing one-hundred-pound weight loss over the period of three years.

Marlon Ransom, former owner of several personal training studios in Chicago, is a certified trainer, a regular contributing writer to various health magazines, and a sought-after speaker on the topics of sales and fitness. He has been friends with Dallas for over a decade and reluctantly took a yoga class at Dallas's behest years ago. Ever since that day, he has been a willing yoga participant and believes in Yoga for Regular Guys as much as Dallas himself.

Cody Runnels always enjoyed competing in amateur wrestling, but it was not until a late-night "gut-check" conversation with DDP that he enjoyed winning in amateur wrestling. While visiting Dallas in Los Angeles, he was introduced to YRG, and as the saying goes, "there was no turning back." He went undefeated during his junior season at Lassiter High School. Athletes and sports commentators alike have always spoken of the importance of being in a "zone," and for Cody, YRG is a one-way ticket there.

RESOURCES

www.diamonddallaspage.com
Here you will find information about Diamond Dallas
Page and his wrestling, acting, and inspirational
speaking careers. Most importantly, you will find
everything you still want to know about YRG. Don't
forget to purchase our YRG workouts on DVD! It's
the perfect workout companion to the at-a-glance
sections and has many fantastic yoga-babe bonuses!

Services

Yoga-Doc
Dr. Craig S. Aaron
2000 Powers Ferry Road, Suite 1-10
Marietta, GA 30067
(770) 859-9579
www.yoga-doc.com

Contact the Yoga-Doc for more information about
power yoga and sports chiropractic, as well as products that will help maintain fitness and health.

Dr. Norman Walker, juicing expert
Norwalk Press
107 N. Cortez, Suite 200
Prescott, AZ 86301
(602) 445-5567

According to Dr. Walker, fruits and veggies have their
own incredible healing and revitalizing properties, but
when mixed in specific recipes and in specific quanti-
ties, they become even more powerful. Dr. Walker's
research has found that juicing can be instrumental in
dissolving gallstones, arterial plaque, and kidney
stones, as well as shrinking and/or preventing certain
types of tumors.

Products

5 Square Low-Carb Meals, by Monica Lynn
(Regan Books, 2004)
www.5squares.com

The key to getting in shape or staying in shape is to
eat high protein and low carbohydrates. Monica Lynn's
5 Square Low-Carb Meals is a cookbook full of plenty
of great-tasting low-carb meals.

Polar Company heart rate monitor
www.polar-heartrate-monitors.com

Most heart monitors have the same working parts.
Just purchase the most basic heart monitor you can
find. The Polar Company makes a very good one.

Ezekiel 4:9 Cinnamon Raisin Bread
Food for Life Baking Company, Inc.
2991 East Doherty
Corona, CA 92879
1-800-797-5090
www.food-for-life.com

Ezekiel 4:9 is not your regular type of bread. It looks
like regular bread, but it is actually 100 percent flourless, sprouted whole grain bread. It's a complete protein, and it's absolutely delicious. The Ezekiel
Company makes and sells all types of flourless
breads, and yes, they are all great. Try Whole Foods,
Trader Joe's, or whatever health food store you have in
your area.

Country Choice certified organic multigrain hot cereal
www.countrychoicenaturals.com

Norwalk Juicer
808 South Bloomington
Lowell, AR 72745
800-643-8645
479-770-0130
www.norwalkjuicers.com

This is the juicer recommended by Dr. Walker's
research institute. It's the mack daddy.

Hyalgan
For more information, talk to your physician or go to
www.hyalgan.com

This is a secret that you may not know about. Hyalgan
is truly oil to this tin man's knees. Hyalgan (pro-
nounced HI-al-gan) is a natural hyaluronan that is
used for patients with osteoarthritis of the knee.
That's the type of arthritis where you develop bone
spurs and wear the cartilage down in your joints. If
you can't get adequate pain relief from simple
painkillers, exercise, or physical therapy, then you
might want to check this out. It is a sterile, highly
purified mixture that is chemically similar to the
hyaluronan normally found in the knee joint.

INDEX

Page numbers in **bold** indicate photographs of specific poses.

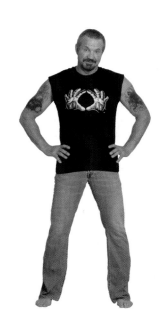